THE ECZEMA HANDBOOK

THE ECZEMA HANDBOOK

A guide to the causes, symptoms
and treatments

Jenny Lewis
with the National Eczema Society

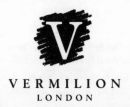

VERMILION
LONDON

Although every effort has been made to ensure that the contents of this book are accurate, it must not be treated as a substitute for qualified medical advice. Always consult a duly qualified medical practitioner. Likewise, you must not regard the suggestions as a substitute for qualified medical advice. Neither the Author, the Publisher nor the National Eczema Society can be held responsible for any loss or claim arising out of the use, or misuse, of the suggestions made or the failure to take medical advice.

First published 1994

1 3 5 7 9 10 8 6 4 2

Copyright © Jenny Lewis 1994

Jenny Lewis has asserted her right to be identified as the author of this work in accordance with the Copyright, Designs and Patents Act 1988.

First published in the United Kingdom in 1994 by Vermilion an imprint of Ebury Press
Random House
20 Vauxhall Bridge Road
London SW1V 2SA

Random House Australia (Pty) Limited
20 Alfred Street, Milsons Point, Sydney,
New South Wales 2061, Australia

Random House New Zealand Limited
18 Poland Road, Glenfield,
Auckland 10, New Zealand

Random House South Africa (Pty) Limited
PO Box 337, Bergvlei, South Africa

Random House UK Limited Reg. No. 954009

A CIP catalogue record for this book is available from the British Library

ISBN: 0 09 178377 1

Typeset in Century Old Style by Textype Typesetters, Cambridge
Printed and bound in Great Britain by Mackays of Chatham Plc Kent

Papers used by Ebury Press are natural, recyclable products made from wood grown in sustainable forests.

CONTENTS

FOREWORD

Eczema is a very individual disease. One person's experience of the condition is not necessarily the same as another's and certainly treatment varies considerably from person to person. However, most people with eczema experience, at some time in their lives, feelings of isolation, rejection, frustration and despondency and these feelings are very often echoed in their families.

This book aims to address that. It has been written, not only to help people manage eczema through medical treatments and environmental factors, but also to acknowledge and discuss the feelings and experiences that are part of the condition.

The Eczema Handbook is not a medical book. It is written in straightforward, easy to read language from the point of view of people with eczema and their carers.

Jenny Lewis joined the National Eczema Society in 1979 because her son had severe eczema and they both found benefit from the Society: Jenny from the practical information and support provided, and Simon from attending the National Eczema Society Children's Holiday Scheme. Jenny has brought much of her own experience to bear in researching and writing this book.

The experiences described by many other members of the Society will undoubtedly strike a chord with most of you. You will see that although the physical condition varies greatly, the emotional experiences are amazingly similar among our members.

Read the book as a comprehensive guide to managing eczema as well as following the daily management routines which include the correct use of essential creams and ointments. The book also discusses how you may be able to control the flare-up of eczema through being aware of the effects of the environment, the role of diet, how to handle stress, how to minimise the scratching and so on.

The more you know about eczema, the better you will be able to keep a sense of balance so that people with eczema and their families can lead full and happy lives, despite the impact of eczema.

Christina Funnell
Director, National Eczema Society
1.2.94

1

WHAT IS ECZEMA?

To a person with a severe form of the condition, eczema is the stuff that nightmares are made of. The parents of an eczematous child will have their lives turned upside down in a round-the-clock routine of bathing, creaming and bandaging while keeping the house, bedding and clothes scrupulously clean and dust free. Through all this they will watch helplessly while the child scratches and bleeds and cries, maybe a little more this day and night but hopefully a little less the next.

The adult will find that the condition separates him from the next man – the latter being the one who is left in peace to get on with his life.

For many people the worst part of the illness is that it is so intensely isolating. People with severe eczema will often hardly leave the house because they cannot bear to be stared at or sometimes ridiculed. It is not unusual for people with this condition to be physically separated from their loved ones because their skin is so raw that they cannot bear to be touched. As teenager, Shelley, explains in Chapter Six: "I would long for a cuddle from my mum and dad, but this wasn't possible as it was just too painful." Perhaps a more fitting name for the illness would be 'Why Me?' – rather than 'atopic eczema', or 'atopic dermatitis', both of which refer to the same condition.

Technically speaking, eczema is a Greek word meaning 'to boil over' – which is how some people feel during a frenzied bout of itching, scratching and trying not to. *Dermatitis* means 'an inflammation of the skin' and since eczema is a problem of the skin perhaps it's worth a brief look at this, the largest organ of the body.

· *The skin* ·

The skin's job is to protect the internal organs from the hazards of the outside world and to contain these organs and keep the body fluids from oozing out. Severe second- and third-degree burns can be fatal and a child who has received burning to just 30 per cent of his or her skin may not survive. A person who has severe eczema may suffer the effects of skin damage. Water loss through damaged skin is just one effect. So if you find that you, or your eczematous child, are drinking a lot, this is to make up the loss of fluid and should be encouraged. (We are talking about non-alcoholic liquid here!)

Equally, if the eczema is widespread it can impair the temperature control functioning of the skin and you can find that you fluctuate between feeling too hot and too cold. The skin regulates temperature by increasing or decreasing blood flow through the blood vessels. In hot weather, when the blood-flow method does not cool down the body quickly enough, the sweat glands help out. When this mechanism is not working well enough, as can happen with eczema, the patient can feel much colder than normal in the extremities (nose, fingers and toes). Also it is thought that people with eczema experience decreased sweating which contributes to the dryness of the skin and the nerve-racking itchiness. Fortunately, both the water loss and the temperature control situations are temporary and improve as the eczema improves.

The skin is made up of two main layers. The top or outer layer is the *epidermis* which in itself is made of several layers. The topmost layer is known as the *stratum corneum*. This is the scaly part that sheds and is constantly replaced by new cells. In the bottom layer of the epidermis are cells known as the *melanocytes*. It is these cells that produce skin pigmentation and determine your skin colour and your ability to tan. Again, eczema has an effect. If the cells are damaged the level of pigmentation they produce changes, sometimes producing increased pigmentation which makes the skin look darker. At other times eczema can cause the melanocytes to temporarily stop pigment production which has the opposite effect. Both these situations are reversible.

Lying underneath the epidermis is the *dermis*. This contains nerve fibres and blood vessels. Nerve fibres produce sensation while the blood vessels do the fetching and carrying of nutrients to the skin. They also play a part in temperature control. Sweat glands and *sebaceous* (oil) glands also appear in the dermis as do the *hair follicles*. *Collagen* and other elastic fibres which appear in the dermis give the skin its elasticity and pliability. As we grow older we have less collagen and elastic fibres in our skin which is why it loses its elasticity and also its resilience.

There are several different kinds of eczema. The most common in children is *atopic eczema*. About one in ten children will develop it at some time in varying degrees of severity. Having said this, atopic eczema can continue into adulthood and can sometimes appear for the first time in adults. Since it is so widespread, the major part of this book is devoted to atopic eczema, although other types of the condition are also covered.

2

ATOPIC ECZEMA

Atopic eczema usually starts in childhood. It can appear as early as the first week of life and tends to improve as the child grows older, but this is not always the case. It can also appear for the first time in adolescence or adulthood. There is usually a family history of eczema or one of the allied atopic conditions – *asthma, allergic rhinitis* and *hayfever*.

It might interest you to know that it is thought that as many as a third of all people will prove to be atopic if tested. Obviously not all of these people will have eczema: many will not experience any of the other atopic illnesses either, but what they all have in common is a predisposition to these conditions.

So if you have a child with eczema and there seems to be no sign of it in your respective families, bear in mind a predisposition to it almost certainly exists.

Atopic people tend to make larger than usual amounts of antibodies called *immunoglobulin E* (or *IgE*). Antibodies exist to defend the body against foreign substances, also known as *allergens*. When these antibodies meet up with undesirable substances, they react, and in the case of eczema this reaction causes inflammation and itchiness.

There are ways of testing people to see if they are atopic by finding out if the patient's body is over-producing IgE. The simplest method is by means of a prick test usually carried out on the inside of the forearm. A tiny drop of a known allergen is introduced into the skin through a needle. If the body reacts it produces a weal. The size of the weal can be measured to give an indication as to how much IgE has been produced to fight the allergen.

Incidentally, allergens can be external substances like pollen, dust, chemicals and so on, or internal, as in the case of food and drink.

· *Recognising the condition* ·

How do you recognise whether or not you or your child has atopic eczema? There are features of this condition which distinguish it from others, but it is most important that you consult a doctor even if you are convinced that the condition is atopic eczema. You should get the condition medically diagnosed and recorded.

· *Indications of atopic eczema* ·

Dry skin

Perhaps one of the most distinguishing features is an excessively dry skin which is also very sensitive. There may be a rash with little blisters or itchy red patches on the fronts of the forearms, behind the knees and on the calves. These common sites of the condition are a very good way of determining whether it is atopic eczema or not.

When the dryness of the skin becomes extreme it cracks open which is both uncomfortable and disabling. When it happens on the backs of the knees it is difficult to walk. It also makes movements painful at the inside of the elbows or the back of the neck. The skin may crack at the sides of the mouth, making it almost impossible to talk.

When I used to meet my son from school he would often be walking awkwardly towards me, looking very strained, and ignoring anyone who greeted him along the way. It meant that he hadn't had easy access to his creams at school and needed to use the emergency supply in my car to lubricate his skin before he could walk properly, or talk. And if I had forgotten to bring the emergency supply with me, we had a very uncomfortable and silent journey back home. It is small wonder that one of the common features of eczema is irritability and surprising that a lesser one is depression.

Red skin – wet eczema

Redness of the skin is another noticeable feature. The medical word for this is *erythema* and it is caused by an increased flow of blood to the skin which in turn has been triggered by an allergen, stress or any of the many triggers that affect a person with eczema. The increased blood flow is accompanied by leaking in the walls of the blood vessels and fluid seeps into the skin.

Scaly skin

In addition to being dry, the skin in a person with eczema is also scaly, although people without any visible signs of eczema can also have a dry, scaly skin. This type of skin condition is inherited and it is thought that people with it may have a predisposition to eczema.

Lichen-like skin

Another recognisable feature of eczema is *lichenification*, where areas of the skin have been constantly scratched or rubbed until the skin thickens and looks leathery. It is given this name because the skin is said to resemble lichen (a microscopic, crusty looking plant-form). The skin can also become darker in colour where there is increased pigmentation. The most common areas for this to appear are the back of the neck, forearms, navel, small of the back, shins and the genital area.

Other features

There are other factors besides skin condition. As we said in Chapter 1, people with atopic eczema will often feel colder in the extremities and be more sensitive to sudden temperature changes. This can trigger bouts of scratching. You become aware of your skin and that can set off the itch and resultant scratching.

When the eczema is severe and the skin inflamed there is a rapid flow of blood to the skin to keep it warm. The heat control mechanism, which normally shuts down the blood flow to the skin to keep the centre of the body warm, is not working. So, initially, when you are exposed to the cold you may not feel it. In fact you may be less likely to feel cold straight away than someone who does not have eczema. But what is actually happening is that your core body temperature is dropping without you being aware of it. And this puts you at a greater risk of getting *hypothermia*, particularly if you have widespread eczema.

Here are some other points to look for:

● Watch the bath water temperature. An eczematous person will not be able to tolerate as hot a bath as other members of the family. Tepid baths are much better.

● Check the water temperature in swimming baths. (We talk about chlorine in Chapter 4.) If your son or daughter with eczema says that the water is too cold for them, take their word for it. Other parents may tell you that their children soon get used to it, but for physiological reasons yours may not be able to adapt. It's nothing to do with guts and courage. People with eczema are almost always very courageous. They have to be!

● Remember about sweating. People with eczema do not sweat as easily as other people, so don't think "they can't be that hot" because they are not sweating. In fact, they may be *very* hot because

of their diminished ability to cool down through sweating.
● Cold weather can make the skin dry and chapped which can exacerbate the eczema.

· *Triggers* ·

Defining triggers and keeping them at bay is covered in other chapters of this book (see Chapter 9 *Keeping Eczema at Bay)*, but here are some of the most common triggers.

Food

This is much more likely to affect children with eczema than adults or adolescents so it is covered in detail in the chapters dealing with babies and children. However, there are some points that need considering in general:

● Don't go on elimination diets or cut out important foods without medical collaboration, either with your doctor or a qualified dietitian.
● Dairy food is very important for children but remember calcium is necessary for adolescents and adults too. So if you are cutting out an important nutrient from one type of food you may need to get it from another, or in the form of a supplement.
● Keep to as varied a diet as you possibly can. If you have a very restricted diet you could find yourself becoming allergic to the foods you eat.

House dust mites

These microscopic creatures eat human skin scales and an eczema person, who produces more scales than others, is particularly attractive to these creatures and house dust mites can present a real nuisance to the eczema patient. They abound in mattresses, settees and carpets and although it is very unlikely that you will be able to eliminate them from your home altogether, you can certainly cut down on their nuisance value by the methods suggested in Chapter 9.

Pets

Lovely though they are, dogs, cats, horses, rabbits and other furry animals can trigger eczema. It is the shed skin, known as *dander*, from the body of the animal, that causes the allergy. Cats are particularly suspect in a house with an eczema patient, but dogs and other animals can also trigger the condition.

Pollens

Grass pollens in particular are anathema to people with eczema. Grasses pollinate in Britain from the beginning of May to the end of July, so sitting on grass or playing sport on grass could be a real problem at this time. Trees pollinate in April and May. (See Chapter 9.)

Stress

A trigger for many illnesses, stress can hardly be avoided, but you can learn to deal with it. (See Chapters 7 and 14.)

Moulds

The spores from moulds and algae can cause allergic reactions in people with eczema. These spores exist in rooms with rising damp but can also live on plants, trees and compost heaps. (See Chapter 9.)

Herpes

People with atopic eczema are particularly susceptible to the virus *herpes simplex* which appears in the form of cold sores, usually around the mouth. However, with someone who has eczema, the virus can also appear on affected areas of the skin and spread quite rapidly, particularly if the eczema is severe. This can lead to a serious condition of eczema known as *eczema herpeticum* (see Chapter 11). You should try and avoid physical contact with anyone with a cold sore as the infection is very easily passed from one person to another, especially babies.

Hygiene

It is important to be fussy about hygiene if you have eczema. In most families, people will sometimes drink from each other's cups, finish off a goody from someone else's plate and may borrow another person's towel. Usually you can get away with all this with no worries. But remember that a person with eczema is much more vulnerable. So don't drink from other people's cups or glasses and don't share towels. If your child has eczema, obviously the same warnings apply. It is a very difficult balancing act you have to perform in giving your child this kind of extra protection and yet keeping him or her from feeling different or ostracised (see Chapters 4 and 14).

Please remember that this book is intended to help you manage the eczema better, maybe even *much* better, but it cannot prevent occasional flare-ups. When they happen try and take them as they come and don't drive yourself mad wondering what you did wrong. Remember that your eczema, or your child's eczema, is not your fault!

3

Babies who have Eczema

There are different skin disorders some of which can start very early on in life, such as cradle cap.

· *Cradle cap* ·

This thick scurfy scalp can appear soon after birth or when the baby is a few months old. It can develop quite suddenly. The scalp becomes coated with greasy yellow scales that stick to the head giving a crusty appearance. This scaliness can affect other parts of the baby's face and head including the forehead, temples, eyebrows, behind the ears and in the neck folds. The skin underneath the scales may look sore, but it is not a condition that causes discomfort or itching and baby will feed and sleep as normal.

During the first few weeks the condition is usually due to the continuing secretion of the greasy coating seen on babies straight after birth. When this dries up the scalp clears.

If the cradle cap develops later on it may be due to *infantile seborrhoeic eczema* and is usually seen on other parts of the body such as the groin and under the arms. *Psoriasis* can also look like cradle cap in infancy as it also causes a scurfy scalp.

If the cradle cap doesn't seem to be clearing up consult your doctor of health visitor. If your baby has accompanying symptoms such as diarrhoea, vomiting or fever, or if he or she is fretful, listless and is not feeding properly, see your doctor straight away. These symptoms may be an indication of psoriasis or seborrhoeic eczema which need a different form of treatment. Or, of course, they can be symptoms of other illnesses and should always be medically checked out.

Treatment

If your baby is diagnosed as having cradle cap, the first thing to know is that you don't actually have to treat it. It is not doing the baby any harm and will go away of its own accord. But if you find it unsightly you can try the following to speed things up:

● Shampoo gently to remove the crust and excess scales. Wash the scalp daily, using a mild baby shampoo and tepid water, but make sure you rub very gently.

● Massage the baby's scalp using slightly warmed olive oil. Again, make sure you work the oil into the scalp very gently. Leave the oil on for an hour or two and then wash off with a mild shampoo. Alternatively, you could massage emulsifying ointment or aqueous cream into the scalp, leave it on for a few hours and wash off with warm water. These creams mix well with water so you don't need to use shampoo as you do with olive oil. If the ointment seems too solid, stand the jar in a bowl of warm water to soften it a little. Be careful not to apply too much pressure as you massage, and pay extra attention to the fontanelle (the soft part at the centre of the baby's head). You can do this daily until the scalp clears.

· *Infantile seborrhoeic eczema* ·

This condition can appear quite suddenly between two weeks to six months after birth. You may notice it first on the nappy area, but it can start on the scalp, or be on both areas at the same time. Once it starts it seems to gather momentum and you may find that it has quickly spread and is on the scalp, face (often including the forehead, temples, eyebrows and behind the ears), neck, armpits, nappy area and the trunk. The good news is that it improves almost as quickly as it spreads! Also, it looks worse than it is. It is not a very itchy condition, nor is it sore. The baby feels well and will eat, sleep and play normally.

Seborrhoeic eczema on the scalp appears in the form of large, yellowy, greasy scales which stick to the scalp making it look crusted. This is why it is often mistaken for cradle cap.

What causes the condition is unknown. Family history of skin conditions does not seem to play a part; nor does it mean that it is going to turn into atopic eczema or another skin condition. The baby may go on to get atopic eczema but it is not related. One in ten children under the age of five have atopic eczema: some of these will have had seborrhoeic eczema as well.

A certain type of yeast has been found on infants who have seborrhoeic eczema and this may be the cause of the rash. But please note that this is not caused by yeasts in the baby's diet.

In its mild form, seborrhoeic eczema is unlikely to become infected. As long as the skin is unbroken it should not cause any problems and is easy to treat. You would be right in suspecting a bacterial infection if the baby's skin feels hot, smells odd, or is weepy. This is most likely to occur in the folds of skin. You need to see your doctor if this happens.

Also the skin may become raw and sore, particularly in the nappy area, and become infected by a yeast called candida which live on the skin in that part of the body. This can lead to thrush. There are creams available to treat severe cases of this condition.

Treatment

● Bathe the baby daily but don't use soap or bubble bath as both of these dry the skin. You can use a soap substitute like aqueous cream, or emulsifying ointment which you can obtain from chemists'. Gently rub the cream or ointment on to the damp skin and then wash it off in the bath. You can also get special bath oils to help moisturise the skin. Please be extra specially careful as the baby will be very slippery!

● Moisturise the baby's skin all over with an aqueous or moisturising cream. Do this several times a day to keep the skin soft and supple. If the skin is sore in places, your doctor may prescribe a weak steroid cream – with 1 per cent (or less) hydrocortisone. Use this sparingly and only in the areas where the skin is sore. If the skin is infected the doctor may prescribe a cream that contains an antibiotic as well as a mild steroid. In the case of thrush the special cream prescribed may be a formula containing an anti-yeast with the steroid. All these creams should only be applied, in small quantities, to the areas infected.

● If it is crusty or scaly, treat the scalp in the same way as cradle cap described above. Again, if the scalp is very sore, your doctor may prescribe a mild steroid cream to use sparingly until the condition improves.

● Change nappies frequently and keep the nappy area clean and dry. This should prevent the skin becoming sore and infected. You may need to change the nappy every hour and you certainly need to change them as soon as they become wet or soiled. If the nappy is wet or soiled, wash the area in a little warm water with oil or cream added. At every nappy change apply an aqueous cream or zinc and castor oil cream to keep the skin soft and protected. Try not to use plastic pants over nappies as they can create hot and humid conditions which help the bacteria breed and can make the eczema worse.

These treatments are time consuming and can be very tiring, but if the baby's skin is sore and infected this extra attention is necessary to help the healing process.

· *Atopic eczema* ·

This condition can develop at any time. It is far more distressing than cradle cap or seborrhoeic eczema because it is itchy and sore. It can appear anywhere on the body, often starting on the face when the baby is three or four months old. The cheeks can become very red and sore, and it then migrates to other parts of the body. The eczema is usually particularly apparent in the body folds; in the backs of the knees and creases of the elbows, on the wrists, ankles, neck, ears and nappy area. It also appears on the eyelids and scalp. One early tell-tale spot is in the place where the ear lobes join the face. If this spot looks at all sensitive, suspect eczema and be careful when you dress and undress the baby. It is very easy to split that part of the skin when you are removing clothing.

Atopic eczema is a dry, scaly, inflamed skin condition. When it is hot the skin dries and cracks open. It is important not to let the baby get too hot or cold. Make sure the bath water is tepid. A baby with eczema does not have the same temperature control as babies without this condition (see Chapter 2).

The severity of the eczema can be very different from baby to baby. One will just have a mild rash say, on the elbows and knees with sensitive or cracking earlobes while another will be covered with an itchy, red, sore and weepy skin and obviously in constant discomfort.

How do you tell if your baby has eczema? Here are some guide-lines but please note that the following is just an indication and you really do need to get a diagnosis from your doctor.

Indications of atopic eczema in babies

● Itchiness is a strong factor but babies tend to rub more than scratch. Look out for redness in the forehead and the wrists as well as cracking and breaking of the skin.
● A dry skin is very indicative of atopic eczema.
● If the eczema is infected it will be weeping and oozing and there may be yellow/brown crusting.

Treatment

You cannot stop a baby rubbing or scratching and you should never make any attempt to tie a baby's hands or restrict movement as this would add to the baby's stress and could make the eczema worse. But you can lessen the effects of the rubbing or scratching by:

● Keeping the baby's nails short
● Covering the baby's hands with cotton mitts or the glove part of

the babygro. Alternatively, you can put cotton socks over the hands having taped the socks to a long sleeved garment the baby is wearing.

● Using cot bumpers can ease the effects of rubbing.

Cutting down on the itch factor is always a question of keeping the skin moisturised and as free as possible from secondary infection by means of special baths.

Bathing babies

Bath babies daily in a bath of tepid water to which a special oil or emollient has been added. Emollients are ointments or creams which are mixtures of water, waxes, fats and oils in varying proportions and they can come in the shape of ointments and creams. Ointments are greasy; creams are not. Ointments are better on a very dry skin so you may want to use that at night, with cream for the daytime. Emulsifying ointments and creams are not as easy to disperse throughout the bath as oil, but you can add a tablespoonful of emulsifying ointment to boiling water and mix these together first, in a separate container, before adding them to the bath.

If the baby is fretful during bath times add lots of toys to the bath as playing with them will help extend the bath and hence the treatment time. But remember never to leave a baby unattended in the bath, and don't forget that he or she will be very slippery when you come to take him or her out.

● Never use soap or bubble bath which dries the skin.

Emollients are safe to use and rarely cause allergic reactions, but products containing lanolin, which is a fat derived from sheep's wool, can occasionally have this effect. It really is a question of trial and error to find out which products suit your baby best.

Bath oils and emulsifiers

Alpha Keri Bath Oil (contains lanolin and fragrance)
Oilatum Emollient (contains lanolin and fragrance)
Aveeno Oilated
Balneum (contains fragrance)
Balneum Plus (contains fragrance)
Emulsiderm
Bath E45

Products to use instead of soap

Aveeno Bar Oilated
Aveeno Bar
Immuderm Body Wash
Neutrogena
Sebamed
Wash E45

Moisturising

Moisturising the skin is very important as it keeps it supple and less likely to crack. You will need to do this at least twice a day, using emollient cream. After the bath is a good time as the skin is moist. Pat the skin with a soft towel leaving it slightly damp. First apply any steroid creams or ointments you have been prescribed, allow time for the medication to be absorbed and then gently apply the emollients.

Always wash your hands before applying creams or ointments and make sure that containers are closed tightly straight after use. Eczematous skin can become infected if the contents of the container are contaminated. If you have more than one eczema person in the family make sure each has his or her own supply of emollients to avoid cross-infection.

Apply cream thinly and smooth it in. If the preparation is thick, apply it in small dots on the parts of the body affected, working from the head to the toes, so the cream will have melted and become more manageable by the time you come to gently smooth it in.

In addition to knowing the names and purposes of the different creams you will be using, it is useful to record how much cream you are using. It usually comes in the following weights: 15gms, 30gms, 50gms or 100gms. Note how many tubes or tubs you use and compare it with the guide below provided by the National Eczema Society.

Minimum amount of emollient cream (gms) required for twice-daily application for one week.

Age	Whole Body	Trunk	Both Arms and Legs
6 months	35	15	20
4 years	55	20	25

Treating with topical steroids

The word 'topical' means something that you apply at the site of the problem. Steroids are substances produced by the body to help the healing process. Steroids produced for medicinal purposes aim to have the same effect. They can be very helpful in treating all manner of illnesses, but taken orally (by mouth) they can have serious side effects, one of which is to restrict growth. This is very unlikely to happen with steroid formulations applied to the skin, but having said that, bear in mind that a baby's skin is very permeable. This is why steroid creams and ointments prescribed for babies are usually of a very weak formulation (1 per cent hydrocortisone) unless there is a special reason for the extra strength – in which case the treatment is likely to be only for a short time. Also, strong doses of steroids used over a length of time can produce thinning, stretch marks and reddening of the skin.

However, topical steroids can reduce itchiness and speed up healing so they are extremely useful in controlling a flare-up of the condition. Used with caution, they can often spare both the baby and parents undue suffering.

If the eczema becomes infected you must see your doctor straight away. Infected eczema can be tricky to treat on anybody, but a baby obviously has to be very closely monitored.

· *Breastfeeding* ·

Breastfeeding seems to be best for the eczematous baby, if it is practical, although research is still a little hazy on this. Firstly, allergy to foodstuffs is not the only trigger. People can be triggered by all sorts of outside allergens including the house dust mite, pollens, animal dander and so on (see in Chapter 2). Also some research studies have found that food allergens can actually be introduced through the mother's milk. If mum is drinking cow's milk, some of the cow's milk protein will be passed on to the baby and although this is in microscopic amounts, it can be enough to induce sensitivity. This is also true of other food stuffs.

So many breastfed babies do get eczema, but breastfeeding may reduce the risk. It is not uncommon for babies to develop eczema soon after being weaned. So if you can breastfeed, do so for the first four months and if you can continue for longer it could help to carry on the protective effect. But remember that breast milk alone is not enough for babies over six months. Your baby will need other foods too.

· *Bottlefeeding* ·

The trouble with campaigns to promote breastfeeding and slogans like 'Breast is Best' is that they can give rise to deep and painful feelings of failure. Many women cannot breastfeed. This is not a particularly modern phenomenon: wet nurses go back a long time.

Motherhood lasts a very long time: breastfeeding accounts for a minuscule portion of it. Mother-love – that special bonding we all need to grow emotionally and become happy human beings – is a million times more valuable than breast milk. There are so many goodies you can offer your baby apart from your breast. An eczematous baby who is lovingly cared for by his or her parents will feel wanted and loved and you can't give better than that.

If you feel that baby's eczema is being triggered by normal formula feeds, there are special formulations you can switch to, but this must be done in consultation with your doctor, dietitian or health visitor. Older children can be switched to a diet that eliminates cow's milk.

Protein hydrolysate formula

This is a special formula where proteins that can produce allergic reactions have been altered. Fats, carbohydrates, vitamins and minerals are added to make the milk similar to human milk in its nutritional content. *Pregestimil*, *Nutramigen* or *Peptijunior* are brand names. As these products are anything but tasty they need to be introduced early on before the baby has developed a taste for flavours!

Soya milk

This is made from soya beans and contains no cow's milk protein. It is nutritious and reasonably tasty but it does have a peculiar smell. Very young children may not notice the smell, particularly if they are drinking it through a nursing bottle or trainer cup. Older children may find it more difficult to get used to. For an adequate calcium supply the child must have at least half a pint a day.

There are two types of soya milk available:

Soya formula milk is a powder formulated especially for babies and young children. It is 'modified' which means that the balance of fats, proteins, carbohydrates and salt is altered to resemble human milk. It is nutritionally complete having had a wide range of vitamins and minerals added, including calcium. Many brands are available from chemists' shops including *ProSobee* (Mead Johnson),

Infasoy (Cow & Gate) and *Wysoy* (Wyeth).

Ready-to-drink liquid soya milks which older children can happily take are available in health food shops and supermarkets. The problem with these is that *they do not contain adequate calcium* so on their own are not sufficient substitute for cow's milk. But they are nutritious in other ways and so long as alternative calcium sources are found, they can be very useful.

However, soya milk can cause allergic reactions in some children in which case you will need to try an alternative.

Goat's milk

Never give goat's milk to a baby under six months of age. Milk has to be modified before being fed to a baby of this age. Goat's milk is not modified, nor is much of it pasteurised (heat treated) and the bacteria can cause lethal infection in infants.

Goat's milk is not subject to the same stringent hygiene controls to guard against harmful bacteria that exist in the production of milk from dairy cattle. Unlike cows, goats are nearly always hand-milked, not machine-milked, and this adds to the risk of contamination.

In addition, many of the proteins in goat's milk closely resemble those in cow's milk, so you may find that changing to goat's milk makes little difference to a child's symptoms.

If you do opt for goat's milk, boil it for at least two minutes. Boiling doesn't improve the taste which is not appealing to everyone in the first place. It also reduces some of the vitamin content, and especially folic acid, which is already low in this milk. By the way, you can supplement the folic acid in your child's diet by giving him or her fresh leafy green vegetables, liver or kidney.

Sheep's milk

This is, to my mind, more tasty than goat's milk but because it is also rarely pasteurised or modified it should be treated with the same caution.

· *Other allergy factors* ·

● *Washing powders or liquids* Although these in themselves do not cause allergy, the biological ones, which contain enzymes, seem to irritate some people's skin more than the non-biological ones do.

Perfume can also be an irritant, so go for non-biological powders or liquids that do not contain enzymes or perfume. Many fabric conditioners also contain perfume so avoid those too. Make sure the garments are thoroughly rinsed so that there is no residual detergent left on them.

● *Wool* Hairy fabrics can aggravate the itch. Cotton is best next to the skin. Viyella is a warmer option and is softer to the touch than wool. In winter you may need to dress a baby in several layers to keep it warm.

● *Clothing* Go for a bigger size as loose-fitting garments are more comfortable. Also make sure that the baby is not overdressed as if he or she gets hot it can make the eczema worse. Look out for other irritants such as rough seams, elastic, labels and metal clips and zips fastenings especially if they are made of nickel.

● *Feathers* Feather duvets and mattresses attract the house-dust mite. Go for man-made fibre fillings in duvets. Cot mattresses are not usually a problem as they are plastic covered anyway.

● *Pets* Household pets shed dander which could trigger eczema or make it worse.

See Chapter 2 and Chapter 9 for further information on triggers.

· *Swimming* ·

More and more parents take their children swimming from a very early age and there is no reason why a baby with eczema should be excluded from this enjoyable activity. As chlorinated water can sting the skin, find out if there is a non-chlorinated pool in your area. Swimming pool water will also dry baby's skin. To remedy this:

● Apply an emollient or barrier cream before going in the pool. (Remember the baby will be slippery but you should be used to this by now!)
● Shower or wash the baby thoroughly after the swim.
● Put more emollient on after drying.

If you get strange glances let people know that your baby has eczema and that it is not catching.

· *A family affair* ·

If your baby with eczema is not your first or only child try not to differentiate between your baby with eczema and the other children in your family. All babies tend to steal the limelight. One who requires extra attention and pulls at your heartstrings can tip the balance much too much. So try and make a point of paying attention to your other children and including them, as much as possible, in the baby's routine. If you don't they will feel neglected and second-best and deep down harbour a resentment that will last long after the eczema has been forgotten. The emotional stress involved, day in day out, can be overpowering. I can tell you that during the years that my son had eczema there were times when I had a very shaky hold on my sanity!

Include everyone in the bathing and creaming routine. An older child could play with the baby and distract him or her while you bathe or cream, but *never* leave your baby in the bath in the care of another child. If they want to help with applying the creams, make sure that their nails are short and very clean.

There is no reason why your other children shouldn't have cream rubbed on their skins or oil in their bath water. It won't do them any harm: quite the contrary. And the baby will grow up feeling the same as his or her siblings.

Explain to all the family what eczema is and that it is not catching. You may feel hesitant about telling people about eczema but your child will often come straight to the point. "That's my brother. He's got eczema. Don't worry you can't catch it!"

Lastly, don't let eczema rule you or your household. Sooner or later there may come a day when the eczema will be gone or very much better. If you have run yourself ragged catering for the baby's every whim you will end up with one dish rag in the house and one small, but tyrannical person.

Handled with sensitivity and understanding, a baby with eczema can be a growing experience for all the family. It can help each member to a deeper understanding of themselves and other human beings.

· *Immunisation* ·

Eczema is not a reason to deny your baby any of the routine immunisations.

The only vaccine that shouldn't be given is the *smallpox* vaccine. People with eczema should never be given this vaccination as serious reactions may develop. It is very unlikely that you will be offered it anyway, since it is no longer required for travel to any country. In the unusual event of you or your child meeting someone who has recently received this vaccine, avoid physical contact. In addition, the vaccinated site should be kept covered until fully healed.

Allergic conditions are not a reason to avoid immunisation (apart from the influenza vaccine which is still cultured on egg and is therefore not suitable for a child who is severely allergic to eggs).

If your baby is unwell, particularly with a temperature, you may be advised to postpone immunisation.

Whooping cough

There has been controversy about this vaccine and perhaps the following pointers will be helpful.

The reasons for having the whooping cough vaccination are:

● Only 1 child in 100,000 has a severe reaction after the immunisation and only 1 in 300,000 suffers brain damage.
● The risk of dying from whooping cough was 1 in 100 in 1940, 1 in 1,000 in 1953, 1 in 5,000 in 1976.

The reasons against having the whooping cough vaccination are, according to the DSS:

● If the child is unwell on the day of the injection.
● If he or she has previously experienced a severe reaction to an injection.
● A history of fits, brain irritation or brain damage in the first 3 months of life.
● Parents or siblings with a history of epilepsy.

These and other worries about the whooping cough vaccine should be discussed with your doctor and individual decisions made in each case.

· *Babies with eczema* ·

Here are the true stories of some babies with eczema. The stories are told by their mothers and I am sure you will find in each of them problems and experiences that relate very closely to yours.

· BABY RIO ·

My three-year-old daughter Rio was born in October 1990. Within a week I was having worries about her skin. She had a slight red rash around her eyes and cheeks. I mentioned this to one doctor who dismissed it as a milk rash or simply the fact that she was unused to wearing clothes! I wasn't satisfied with this diagnosis but left it at that. The rash gradually got worse and at the same time she developed what I thought was bad cradle cap, the crown of her head started to crack and bleed. She was about three weeks old when the health visitor spotted this and commented that she didn't know Rio had eczema.

This was the first time eczema had ever been mentioned to me and I was understandably shocked. I had always thought of eczema as scabs on the joints, never giving a thought to how they got there or why. I immediately took Rio to our G.P. who confirmed this. Since that day life seems to have been one cream, bath oil and bandage after another.

Her skin gradually got worse and worse and when she was about eight months old we started having to use steroid creams all over her twice a day and this has been going on ever since. From that time onwards she has also been taking various syrups to help her sleep.

She is now totally dependent on these sedatives to help her sleep and she rarely sleeps for more than a couple of hours at a time.

I dislike using steroid creams and sedatives over such a long period of time but the doctors repeatedly tell me I have little choice as they are the only effective ways of keeping Rio's eczema under control and making her life bearable.

She spent much of the time between her first and second birthdays bandaged from the neck downwards and she was also admitted to hospital a couple times when she was very down.

There is no doubt that Rio's life has been affected adversely by her skin condition. The skin all over her body is very dry in spite of the various creams and moisturisers. The skin on her joints, stomach, nipples, thighs, hands and toes crack and bleed constantly. This is made much worse by the itching and swelling.

One of the most upsetting things about eczema is the attitude of other people. The way they stare and the hurtful comments they make. One of our worst experiences took place in the doctors' surgery. Rio started to play with two other children when their mother moved them to the other side of the room and told them not to play with her. Luckily Rio was too young to understand the reasons. But we did.

· BABY JAMES ·

James has had eczema since he was three weeks old. He is now 21 months. When he was younger it was on his face and the backs of his knees as well as his arms, neck and trunk. He also had a thick scaly mess on his head. I was a new mum and I didn't know what to do. There wasn't a lot of help around. I kept thinking it was something I was doing that was causing it. Our G.P. kept saying he would grow out of it.

When he gets hot he sweats and then he starts scratching. He has also developed asthma and hayfever. He gets stressed out over the asthma and that brings on the eczema.

They gave me Vallergan Forte *for the night and that did help because he slept and didn't scratch as much. But during the day if he wasn't 'half out of it' he'd be scratching. He could get his mittens off. He could even pull the gloves on his babygro off.*

I didn't like taking him out. He looked awful, with what looked like friction burns on both sides of his face. People would ask me what I'd done to him. I wanted to keep a hat on him all the time to hide his head.

I find the scratching very distressing, especially at night. It's only a one-bedroom flat so he is in the bed next to me. I can hear him scratching. I have to keep getting up to stop him or he'll scratch his face to pieces. A few times he's taken chunks out of his face. It's been awful.

I find the constant creaming and bathing him quite difficult: then there's the washing and drying of the sheets constantly. The scales from his skin, the blood and the creams get all over the sheets. It's expensive keeping him in cotton clothes, but I have to.

I also work part-time and the disturbed nights make this difficult.

· BABY EMILY ·

Emily is two-and-a-half years old. Her eczema started when she was aged about nine months. It's on the crooks of her arms, knees, tops of her feet, her wrists and hands. Between her fingers are the worst places and that's where she most often gets infected, probably because she can't stop herself from scratching. On those places it's the classic eczema – angry red weals. But on the rest of her body there are spots. I'm told it's also eczema but it looks quite different.

She was purely breastfed until she was four months and then everything else was introduced. She went on to a normal diet. I had no reason to put her on to special milks or anything. There was no evidence of the eczema before she was nine months old and neither my husband nor I can trace it in our families. There's no asthma either as far as I am aware, but my sister has hayfever.

At the moment the worst part is the creaming in the morning and evening from head to toe. It always raises absolute hysteria. As soon as she gets cream all over her she wants a cuddle. She's absolutely desperate for a cuddle. We say: "In a moment we'll give you a big cuddle." She gets very upset and launches herself at us which means that we all have grease all over us and have to get changed. It's used for effect. She knows exactly what she's doing. But at the moment it is causing the whole family a lot of stress twice a day.

I get worked up thinking "I can't put it off longer, she's had a bath, I've cleaned her teeth. Now I've got to cream her." I've taken to reading her the bedtime story while I'm putting it on. That's the worst time. She makes a big issue of it and we all know how important it is.

I have tried experiments. About a fortnight ago my mother said to me: "It can't be any worse, why don't you just stop it," and so I did. On her right leg I used nothing. On her right arm, which was particularly bad at the time, I used all the usual stuff plus the 1 percent steroid instead of the 0.5 percent. The rest of the body I treated the same as usual. Within a couple of days the right leg was noticeably worse and the right arm was noticeably better. Not horrendously worse and not cured, but within two days I decided not to carry on the experiment any longer because I thought that the evidence was there.

Over the last six months we've had very little sleep – any of us. She wakes up all the time in spite of the Phenergan. Sometimes we are woken up five or six times in the night. I don't work so I usually get up, but there are occasions when I just can't get up any more, I'm so tired, and my husband has to do it instead.

There was a night last week when she woke up at a quarter past one and I didn't get her to sleep until about six in the morning. I did everything. I did the cuddling, comforting, persuading, distracting and then I got to the screaming and threatening – the worst things you could possibly do, I know, but I was desperate. Then I had to take hold of myself and say: "This is stupid; you are only making things worse for both of you. Take a breather." We played musical bedrooms. She came in with me.

People tell me to sleep during the day when she does. But she doesn't sleep during the day. If she ever does fall asleep I think: "Oh great! I'll do this..."

· NICKY ·
(aged 3)

I breastfed Nicky until he was 10 months old. He'd had skin problems from birth. I gave him a little bit of egg yolk on the suggestion of the health visitor. It was less than a spoonful. Until then he had enjoyed trying the different tastes, but with this he pulled a face and didn't like it. His lips swelled. He cried and the crying was a deep throaty chesty cry which I hadn't experienced before. He was struggling to breathe. His eczema was really bad. It was a nightmare. I had to call an ambulance. By the time he got to hospital the eczema was so bad he had scratched himself to such an extent that he was bleeding. By this time he was very docile and the swelling had gone down. They gave him Piriton *syrup. They kept him there until they felt he was all right, but the hospital staff were so horrified at the extent of his eczema that they suggested we brought him back for treatment.*

Previously I had tried him on one of the formula baby milks and when I'd given him that it had caused an urticaria *around his lips. The health visitor suggested I use* Wysoy *milk which he enjoyed. I didn't give him very much because the doctor said it was better to carry on breastfeeding.*

I don't eat meat although through my pregnancy I did try and eat a bit of meat, but I don't like it. During pregnancy I felt I had to have a balanced diet and I ate a lot of cheese and drank a lot of milk to get the protein. Perhaps I went over the top.

I saw a dietitian who said it would be best to stop breastfeeding him as soon as possible. Funnily enough, he had really bad eczema on his face, but soon after I stopped breastfeeding his face cleared up.

His face was so bad at one time that they recommended using a lot of creams. The use of steroid creams bothered me. I didn't like it, but it was something I had to do. It got to the stage where it was so weepy he was obviously bothered with it. If I took the gloves off his hands he would just scratch his face and I'd feel terrible about it. Everything would be okay and suddenly he'd have this itching fit and his face would just bleed and bleed. I began to wonder what I was doing wrong.

He's on a dairy-free diet now. He can't have white fish either, or ham, and some E numbers make him very high.

When he had it badly, he would scratch dreadfully at night. I'm only just beginning to have some good nights now. When he was a baby I'd end up crying in the night sometimes. I didn't know whether to shake him and go berserk, or what. You feel so alone at night. And he was up a great deal.

I find the Ichthopaste *bandages are wonderful. A few nights of bandages can sometimes stop it getting out of hand. I think that if I left it, the eczema would be out of control, and once you let that happen it's harder to get it back to normal.*

Nicky is getting to the stage where he feels he is different. The birthday parties are difficult because he knows he can't have some of the foods. We've had two parties recently and the people giving them have known the situation and they've been very kind. They've done exactly the same food for everybody, but used the kind of margarine and chocolate he can have, instead of milk chocolate. I've been lucky in that they've gone out of their way to make it easy for me.

I feel there is light at the end of the tunnel because we do experience good times. Now, if we have a little blip, I remind myself that we are just experiencing a bad time and it will pass.

CHILDREN WHO HAVE ECZEMA

We know that *atopic eczema* is a condition that is inherited and depends on body chemistry. We also know that it is not catching. You can share a bed, sleeping bag, bathe or swim with an eczematous person and you won't catch it. But how much of this does your child know? Children are extremely vulnerable to the ignorance of others. Knowing what eczema is and where it comes from is very important to your child. Another child may point to a particularly sore patch on the skin and say, "Ugh – you're dirty!" And your little one may believe this regardless of the constant regime of bathing, dusting and washing clothes. Even adults with eczema say that they feel dirty although they know logically that nothing can be further from the truth.

Some children may feel that it's their fault that they have got a condition like eczema – they've done something wrong, or there is something inferior about them. Having the condition simply explained can go a long way in helping children cope with it. Talk about eczema in an open way and encourage your child and other members of the family to do the same.

Other types of eczema conditions are covered in Chapter 11.

· *Psychological issues* ·

When my son, Simon, was little and his eczema was severe I knew, having joined the National Eczema Society, that there was an odds-on chance that he would grow out of it. What I didn't know was whether or not he would suffer psychological damage which he would carry for the rest of his life. He would come home from school miserable, his skin all cracked and bleeding, and would have to get into a bath while the other children played outside. I silently agreed with him that it wasn't fair! When he fell behind with his school work because his hands were so bad that he couldn't hold a pen, or fell asleep in class because he had been awake all night scratching or was still suffering the effects of sedation, I despaired of him ever getting a normal education. When he couldn't have a dog or a cat, or stroke a horse, or play in the summer grass with the other kids, I thought to myself: "This child is not having a good childhood." It made me worry about his current state of mind and future as an adult.

It is difficult to ensure that a child who has clearly got something different about him feels that he is the same as everybody else. But a child with eczema *has* special needs: he or she will need special help with treatments and avoidance of triggers as well as an extra helping of tender loving care. But more special than that is the need to be the same as everybody else. Here are some do's and don'ts that I think will help. Please note that although I usually use 'him' and 'he' throughout, this book also refers to girls with eczema!

● *Don't make one law for him and another for the other children in the family.* If you give in to unreasonable demands or let your eczematous child get away with things the others don't, you could end up with a rather demanding young person on your hands with an unreal perception of what life is all about. Added to which, he may alienate friends with his behaviour and end up being rather lonely.

● *Ignore the tantrum scratch.* Most people are manipulative given half a chance and children certainly 'try it on'. A child who knows that you are worried about his skin will try using it as a weapon. "If you don't give me what I want I'll hurt myself and that will hurt you" is an often-used bargaining position. Don't punish; let him scratch. It will hurt you. It will hurt your child. But if he doesn't get a reaction it won't happen too often. And he won't start playing psychological mind games every time he doesn't get his own way.

● *Encourage communication.* Many people reach adult life with an inability to share their feelings with others. They have grown up with the impression that they have to keep their thoughts and feelings to themselves for fear of being thought weak and vulnerable. Having feelings is not a sign of weakness; it is normal, as is being vulnerable. A child who has eczema may have some very negative feelings about his or her condition. He may feel he has been 'singled out' for punishment. If he can learn to share these kinds of feelings with family and friends, not only will it ease the burden of the condition, but he will become a much more open and emotionally confident person than many of his non-eczematous counterparts.

● *Don't be over-protective.* Let your child do the same things as siblings and friends unless an activity is particularly harmful. There will be some no-go areas, but try to keep these to a minimum. As long as the eczema is not likely to get too bad or the risks are not too high, give it a chance. There is no point in controlling your child's eczema to the point where it makes him afraid of life.

● *Include siblings.* Put oil in the other children's baths and lotion or cream on them too – it can only benefit their skins. And if you find yourself spending more time cleaning your eczematous child's room than the entire house, don't moan about it within earshot or it will make him feel troublesome and guilty.

● *Take schoolwork seriously.* There will be times when your son or daughter may have to miss school or be less attentive in class because of the eczema. But don't let the eczema become an excuse for not going to school when he doesn't feel like it. There may be types of jobs that your child cannot do because of allergic reactions so you really need to make sure that he gets the best education on offer to give a wide career choice.

● *Give your child responsibility for his eczema wherever possible.* As soon as he can cream himself and run his own baths – encourage him to do it. Make him responsible for keeping his skin clean and putting the tops on the creams and lotions. The more children can do for themselves the greater the confidence they will have about doing different activities – visiting friends, sleeping-over and so on – and the less the eczema will rule your lives.

● *Talk about the condition in the family.* The more everyone understands about the condition the more they will be able to inform others and the less vulnerable they will be to teasing. There is no fun in teasing someone who doesn't react. In the school playground I once heard one boy try to taunt another by saying: "You're very short and you're very fat." The short, fat boy shrugged, looked amazed and somewhat disdainful and said: "I know." His complete indifference to his physical appearance made his taunter feel very foolish and he ran away. If having eczema is treated as normal and unremarkable in the family it will help the child project this attitude to it in the outside world and the condition will be less available for use as a weapon.

The last point to bear in mind is that eczema is unlikely to leave behind psychological scars. Children have short memories and once the skin condition has stopped being a problem, they seem to forget it. For my part, I certainly did not get everything right, yet when I ask my son, now aged 19, about his eczema he says he cannot remember very much about it, and I can see no signs of psychological scarring.

· *Keeping eczema at bay* ·

Much of atopic eczema is about allergies. You inherit a pre-disposition to the condition and various allergens trigger it. There are many possible triggers and they are difficult to avoid. What we can do is list the best known triggers and give some guidance on how to avoid them. Details of the nine most common triggers listed below are given in Chapter 9.

Common triggers of eczema

- House dust mites
- Pets
- Pollen
- Bedding
- Furnishing
- Fungi and moulds
- Washing powders and liquids
- Clothing
- Tobacco smoke

It is better for your child if you can control the eczema through the environmental factors listed above rather than through diet. Not only are strict diets socially inhibiting but they need a great deal of skill and vigilance if they are to work, and expert help if they are to ensure that your child is provided with the nutrition he or she needs.

Having said that, food allergy can contribute to the condition in some children. The younger the child the more likely this is to be so. Studies show that dietary treatment works best in the first few years of life. Adults and older children are not so affected by it.

· Food allergy ·

Finding which foods your child is allergic to is neither simple nor obvious. Sometimes parents think they've tracked it down when they notice that touching a certain food produces swelling of the mouth or wealing on the skin at the site of contact. This is known as *contact urticaria* and although it may seem very alarming, particularly if the whole face swells up, it may be that your child is not allergic to the food once it is swallowed. It may be, for instance, that taking a bite out of a tomato may make the area around the mouth red whereas cut up small in a salad, or skinned and cooked, tomato will have no effect at all. Similarly, your child may not be able to eat oranges as such without causing an allergic reaction, but orange juice taken through a straw may not constitute a problem. The same goes for other acid fruits.

Sometimes foods that affect on contact also have an allergic effect in the body. The effect may not necessarily be eczema. Sometimes the reaction may be that the child complains of a stomach ache or is sick. Other times the skin may break out in weals an hour or so after the food has been eaten; or the skin may become very red and/or very itchy.

These reactions which occur soon after a food has been eaten are known as *immediate hypersensitivity reactions*. Foods that produce these kind of reactions usually come up positive on skin prick tests and *Radio-AllergoSorbent Tests (RAST)* which are carried out with a blood sample. However most dermatologists do not feel that these tests are at all helpful. They can come up positive on food that the child cannot touch without a reaction but can eat quite safely, so there would be no reason to eliminate it altogether from the child's diet. As far as eczema is concerned, there can be a delay of several hours or days between eating a food and a reaction to it occurring. Sometimes the food needs to be eaten often before a reaction occurs and the quantity eaten may be critical too.

The best way to test for food allergy is the hard way – by trial and error. Keeping a diary of what the child eats and noting any reactions is a good idea because it should pin down what affects your child on an individual basis. But the diary will have to be kept assiduously over several weeks, if not months, to be really effective.

· *Diet* ·

There are three important rules to follow in making diet part of your child's long-term eczema prevention plan.

1) Don't do it without collaborating with an expert in the shape of your doctor or dietitian. A growing child has many nutritional needs and if you are excluding an important food – dairy products for instance – you will need to make up for it in other ways.

2) Don't exclude foods 'just in case' or because your friend's child's eczema got better by eliminating a certain food. The most important point to remember is that you should keep your child's diet as varied as possible. People can become allergic to the foods they eat most often. If your child has a very restrictive diet, not only may he be missing out on vital nutrition, but he may become allergic to some of the foods he is currently eating with impunity.

3) Understand that food has social implications. A child who is on a restricted diet will find parties difficult. He may feel discouraged from going to friends' houses where he might be offered food that he cannot eat. Children do daily 'deals' with food-treats at school. My son used to swap his home-made cakes and biscuits for Mars bars as soon as he reached the playground. Needless to say we knew nothing about it until many years later. Some children will co-operate on diets while others will not!

A child whose eczema is very reactive to food may be more inclined to co-operate, particularly if you can narrow it down to one or two foodstuffs. However, since eczema has so many different triggers you may find that eliminating a foodstuff may only improve the eczema marginally. This may not be a good enough incentive to make your child carry the burden of not eating what other children eat and be 'different'. So keep an open mind about it. Also bear in mind that tolerance to food occurs as children grow older, so foods that they are allergic to now may present no problems later on.

Exclusion diets

An exclusion diet for a child will mean cutting out cow's milk and eggs as well as other items. These could be chicken, some food additives and some colouring like *tartrazine (E102)* and certain preservatives like *benzoate* which can aggravate eczema in some cases (see page 39). Nuts, tomatoes and fish can also trigger eczema for some people.

Please do not attempt an exclusion diet on your child without the help and support of both a doctor *and* a dietitian. The doctor can be your G.P., a pediatrician, dermatologist, or a clinical immunologist.

What the doctor can do is to ensure that the diagnosis of eczema is correct and advise on the different kinds of treatment that are available, other than diet. This will include creams, ointments and so on. He or she can also prescribe nutritional supplements like milk substitutes, calcium tablets as well as minerals and vitamins. The doctor can put you in touch with a dietitian who can check on the adequacy of an exclusion diet and advise on any necessary supplements that may be required. The dietitian can also provide lists of suitable and unsuitable foods for your child's diet, help you interpret food labels and also supply you with ideas and recipes for nutritious meals.

If the diet is going to help it will usually do so within six weeks. You will not see the full benefit of the diet if you abandon it too early. Try and explain this to your child so that he understands what it is all about.

If the diet seems helpful the next step is to work out which foods affect the eczema out of all those that have been excluded. To do this you will need to introduce the items one by one. Ideally, a full week should be allowed for each item. With milk, for example, one teaspoonful only should be given on the first day. If no adverse effects follow, give between half a pint and one pint on each of the next six days.

You should not expect to be able to tell whether your child's eczema is aggravated by a food if you only give a small amount from time to time. But bear in mind that the eczema may not develop for a few days after the food has been eaten. At the end of the week, if there has been no change in the eczema, you should not worry about re-introducing milk into the diet on a more permanent basis. If at any time during the week you feel there may have been an unrelated explanation for an adverse reaction, you could try again later.

Every year try to re-introduce foods that are still being excluded from your child's diet. You will often find that the allergic response disappears as the child gets older.

Few-food diets

This is an alternative to the elimination diet and can be used if the former has produced negative results. It is not practised very often these days because it is hard work, very restrictive, particularly for children, and rarely beneficial. But the idea is that an individual may have their eczema triggered by *any* food. So to begin with a very limited number of foods is ingested – maybe only six items. This continues for two to four weeks. If results are good a single item of food is added each week. This way you can isolate what is affecting you and eliminate it altogether from the diet. Eventually you build up a picture of what you can and cannot eat without aggravating the eczema.

This kind of diet has to be carried out under expert supervision, particularly with children. This is not only to ensure that you are getting the nutritional balance right, but also to be certain that you are not inadvertently ingesting other foodstuffs.

· Cow's milk ·

Along with eggs, cow's milk seems to be the most common culprit in aggravating eczema, but it is a very important food for children because it is rich in protein and calcium which is essential for the normal growth of teeth and bones. So if you are contemplating putting your child on a cow's-milk-free diet you will need to supplement the loss of protein with extra meat, fish, pulses and a complete milk substitute. The calcium loss can be replaced with a calcium tablet or with the complete milk substitute such as soya milk, goat's milk or protein hydrolysate (see page 22).

If you are eliminating cow's milk from the diet because you believe it is aggravating the eczema, you have to make a thorough job of it. Just not drinking milk is not enough. You have to avoid cow's milk, cheese, butter, cream, yoghurts, ice cream, milk powders (full-fat and skimmed) and non-fat milk solids and you will need to scan the contents list of everything you buy to make sure that milk protein does not appear in them. There are replacements. There are soya-milk ice creams and sorbets and goat's and sheep's milk cheeses and yoghurts which are absolutely delicious. But excluding milk is difficult which is another reason why expert help is so necessary. *Whey*, for instance, which appears in many margarines and shortening, is a milk protein, as are *casseinates* which seem to be included in many food products. *Lactalbumen* and *lactose* are two other products to look out for and avoid.

· *Soya milk* ·

This is made from soya beans and contains no cow's milk protein. The problem is that it does not contain adequate calcium so on its own is not a sufficient substitute for cow's milk. But it is nutritious in other ways and so long as alternative calcium supplements are found it can be a very useful part of a milk-free diet.

Even so, soya milk can cause allergic reactions in some children in which case you will need to try another alternative.

· *Calcium supplements* ·

If your child is not getting enough calcium through milk it should be supplemented in tablet form. *Sandocal* tablets are good as one dissolved in water or orange juice daily is more than adequate. These tablets contain a very small amount of E102 and E110 food colouring but not in sufficient quantity to cause any problems as a rule. Alternatively you could try Cox effervescent calcium gluconate tablets which contain no added colouring but your child may need to take up to six daily to get an adequate calcium supply.

· *Eggs* ·

Eggs can be eliminated from the diet without risk. Protein can be provided by meat, fish and pulses instead. An egg is a common constituent of ready-made food, so check the labels and contents for dried egg powder, egg yolk, egg white, egg albumin, egg lecithin and ovalbumin.

Egg replacers can be found in health foods. They come under such headings as 'Egg Replacer' or 'Egg-white Replacer' or 'Whole-egg Replacer'. But beware of the phrase 'egg substitutes' as some of them can be based on egg protein. You will need to check food labels regularly and if in doubt, give the item miss.

Chicken is often eliminated along with egg on the basis that it is the same protein and if you are allergic to one you are likely to be allergic to the other. But this isn't always the case and you should bear in mind that the more varied the diet the better it is.

· *Food additives* ·

After milk and eggs, some artificial colouring and some preservatives are the most commonly implicated in eczema. As a rule of thumb, children with eczema should be fed as much as possible with fresh food. Artificial colouring and preservatives appear on labels either by name or their 'E' number. A number without an E before it means that the colour is not permitted at all in some EEC countries.

Not all E numbers are bad and you really should equip yourself with one of the many 'E' number paperbacks that are available these days. They give a great deal of information on additives and are invaluable for this kind of dieting.

The two groups of additives that are thought to most commonly aggravate eczema are the *benzoate preservatives* and the *azo colouring*. There are 10 benzoate preservatives with E numbers used in food: E210 to E219. These can appear in jams, sauces and syrups, cake mixes, drinks, salad cream, pickles, coffee and chicory essence, fruit purée and pulps, glacé fruits and many other. Small amounts of benzoic acid occur naturally but it is the synthetically prepared benzoates added to food that seem to cause the problems.

The most commonly used azo dyes are tartrazine (E102), sunset yellow (E110), amaranth (123) and ponceau (E124). These can appear in smoked food, convenience food, sweets, chewing gum, squash, pickles, sauces, drinks, biscuits, cake mixes, jams, soups, jellies, pie fillings, tinned fruit and others.

Other colourings that may cause problems are: E122 Carmoisine (red colour), E131 Patent Blue, E132 Indigo Carmine, E133 Brilliant Blue, E155 Brown HT.

Unwrapped foods like bread and cakes do not require full labelling nor do chocolate and cocoa products. Needless to say some of these will have food additives in their contents and the only way to find out is to contact the manufacturers direct. Small packages of food need not have ingredients listed.

Many medicines and syrups contain artificial colouring and preservatives as do toothpastes, vitamins and mineral preparations.

None of these need to have their ingredients listed. The chemist may be able to advise you but if not you will need to get in touch with the manufacturer.

· *Other allergies* ·

As you can see, elimination and restrictive diets can be hard work to implement and difficult to keep up, and the older the child is, the less likely food is to play a part in eczema. So it really is advisable to first try and cut down on other possible allergens and only use a diet if those measures are not effective.

By and large these measures are the same whether it is a baby, child, adult or elderly person who has the eczema. So it is covered for everyone in Chapter 9, *Keeping Eczema at Bay*. Please read this chapter for advice on the control of house dust mites, pollens, soaps and detergents, clothing and bedding as well as other allergens that are known to aggravate the condition. However, for children, a special point needs to made regarding pets.

· *Domestic pets* ·

There are many myths about pets and eczema. Cats and eczema don't mix but it has nothing to do with whether the cat has short hair or long hair. The allergic reaction is caused by dander which is the dust from the small scales in the cat's skin. Cats shed dander continuously whether they are of the short-haired or long-haired variety. Cat's urine and dried saliva are also allergenic. If you have a cat, check whether your child's eczema is on the backs of the thighs and the fronts of the knees. If they are, it could be cat-induced. What about your child's face and hands where he has been cuddling the pet – are they affected too? Children with eczema can be very sensitive to cats, if not at first, they may become so later on. And the allergy may take the form of asthma as well as eczema.

Dr Atherton, who has done an enormous amount of work with children with eczema, says that some children become so acutely allergic to cats that they are affected even if they enter a room in which a cat has been a day or so previously. In his book, *Your Child with Eczema* he says: "If your child has eczema, it would be wise to do without a cat. Although I love cats, if you already have one, I would advise you to get rid of it and look out for a friend or relative who is prepared to look after it to save you having to put it down." Dr Atherton adds that it can take several weeks or months for the eczema to start to improve once the cat has gone because it can take that long to get rid of the last traces of the dander. Friends may say to you: "Your daughter strokes the cat when she is in our house and nothing happens." She may get away with it on an occasional basis but a live-in cat could be a very different story!

It is not that different with dogs. Although they seem to be a little less allergenic than cats, they too could be a problem when kept by a family where there is a child with eczema. Again it is the dander so it makes no difference whether the dog is short haired or long haired or whether it is a breed that doesn't shed hair at all. The dog's saliva and urine are again implicated and you may find that your child develops weals on the skin where he has been licked.

No one is denying that pets can add a great deal of fun and emotional enhancement to family life, but you have to weigh that against the possibility that they can aggravate the eczema.

Allergic reactions have been reported from many animals, not just dogs and cats. Birds are implicated and, at the risk of sounding repetitious, I must tell you that it is the dander and droppings that seem to cause the allergy rather than the feathers. Rabbits, guinea pigs and mice can also be a problem for the eczematous child. He may be able to tolerate horses occasionally but if it is a constant relationship an allergy could well develop. Farm animals like sheep, cows and pigs may also pose a problem.

Ever thought about iguanas? Or tropical fish? They may not be quite the same, but alternative pets do exist!

· *Allergy testing* ·

As explained in Chapter 2, there are tests available to find out if a person is atopic. There are tests which try and pinpoint people's allergies. Dermatologists and specialist skin clinics can carry out prick tests where the surface of the skin is broken and a series of known allergens are introduced to see if they cause a reaction. Patch tests, which work in a similar way to detect contact eczema, are also used. But although they can give clues they are not a hundred percent reliable. As we have seen, a person can be allergic to touching a food which gives no trouble at all once it has been eaten.

· *Treatment* ·

The most important part of eczema control is to get into a daily routine of bathing and moisturising the skin. Eczematous skin is dry and porous. You have to counteract that and the way to keep it moisturised is by applying emollients gently and frequently. You must carry on doing it even when the eczema seems to be clear because the skin can look fine when it has not healed entirely underneath. It gets itchy and then gets scratched and the whole thing starts up again.

If the eczema is mild all the child will need is a daily bath to which an oil or emollient has been added. Make sure that the water is warm but not hot. The use of a soap substitute will also be helpful in preventing the skin from drying. Please don't leave a young child alone in the bath, but let him soak there for 15 to 20 minutes. Then moisturise the skin by applying emollient to act as a barrier to keep it from becoming more dry. Should the condition become more severe you will need to supplement this routine with a steroid cream which you use only on the affected parts.

If steroid creams are being used put them on first and give them time to sink in before applying the moisturising cream. This helps to increase absorption of the steroid cream. Try and moisturise the skin at least twice a day. You may also need to give the child an antihistamine tablet to cut down the scratching, particularly at night. And if the eczema becomes infected you will need to contact your doctor to get prescribed a special antibiotic cream to quickly clear up the infection. You may be prescribed an oral antibiotic to clear the infection. Chapter 12 details this daily routine and explains and lists the various topical and oral preparations involved. Antihistamine creams should *not* be used on eczema as they may cause an allergic reaction.

· *Scratching* ·

It's no good telling your child who is currently being driven insane by an overwhelming total body itchiness "Don't scratch!" It's like telling someone who is very unhappy: "Don't cry!" It doesn't make the pain go away. It just adds to the feeling of guilt. What you can do is to protect against scratching and help your child find an alternative relief to the itch. Here are some tips:

● Keep nails short and clean: filing them is better than cutting as the latter leaves sharp edges. You will need to check on nails daily.
● If you can find a distraction so much the better.
● Try and get your child to rub, pat or press the itchy area. It is less destructive than scratching.
● If you can apply an emollient when the itch begins it will help cool

the skin down. Encourage your child to keep a tube of emollient with him to use when the itching starts.
● Protect against scratching at night. You can make socks and mittens out of tubular bandage and tape it to wrists and ankles, or attach it to nightwear.
● Wearing cotton gloves can be helpful during the day.

· *Bandaging* ·

The thought of bandaging a child with eczema can be very off-putting. Some parents won't use bandages at all as they consider them to be hot and itchy. Others bandage their children from head to toe at night for protection and medicated bandages can help with the healing.

● *Tubular bandages* are more effective than ordinary crêpe bandages for protection and can be very useful for making mitts. They come in a wide range of sizes from those that fit little fingers and toes to those that fit a larger child's body. Try not to bandage all over but if you have to, only do it at night.
● *Medicated bandages* are not used so often for children. Soaked in paste (zinc and coal tar and a mild steroid or Ichthopaste) they are used primarily for treating adults with limb and varicose eczema. However, they can be used for children especially if the skin has become very thick and leathery. The tar is grey and messy, so tar bandages are best used overnight under old pyjamas. They have a cooling effect, relieve irritation and speed up healing.

· *Hair and scalp* ·

It is not uncommon for children to have eczema in the scalp but it is usually mild and a suitable medicated shampoo is all they are likely to need. It is best not to leave the child to wash his own hair – better for someone without eczema to do it to avoid possible hand problems. Products containing coal tar are usually effective, but some people are allergic to tar in which case a non-tar shampoo is recommended. If *seborrhoeic eczema* is diagnosed an anti-yeast preparation may be prescribed. Sometimes steroids are used to speed up the process. These will be in mild form used for a short amount of time with children since the skin on the scalp is highly absorbent. Your doctor or pharmacist can suggest suitable shampoos.

· *Antihistamines* ·

Taken orally, antihistamines can be very helpful in treating eczema. They do not cure the condition but they can reduce the scratching. Children have been given quite large doses of antihistamine for many years without there being any evidence that they are either addictive or harmful. Non-sedative antihistamines are not considered to be of any use in treating eczema, so you do need to give the sedative version. Obviously this is best done at night. If you give the dose early enough (at least an hour before bedtime) there is less likely to be a hangover effect in the morning. Obviously you will need advice from your doctor on dosage. But you do need to give a large enough dose to help the child sleep. If there is a hangover effect in the morning in spite of the fact that you administered it early, the dose was probably too high and you will need to cut back.

The body can develop immunity to antihistamines so they can become less effective in some children. For this reason it is worth limiting the use of them. Don't use them if the eczema is mild enough for the child to sleep or not scratch without them. This way they won't lose their efficacy and will be useful as an ally in the bad times.

If your child has been on antihistamines for a time and the condition is now better, withdraw them gradually so that the body gets used to being without them.

If your child is taking the antihistamine in syrup form, brush the teeth after the dose to avoid decay. If you suspect he is allergic to colouring ask for undyed tablets or syrups.

· *Parties and sleep-overs* ·

Parties are, of course, going to offer a hundred-and-one temptations to a child who is on a special diet. With each party invitation comes the dilemma: do you let the child go, knowing that he is going to eat things that will make the eczema worse – or do you refuse, assuring the child that it will be better for him in the long run? Don't agonise about it; let the child go, and cope with the consequences if and when they arise. Don't even saddle the child with a list of what they can't eat. It is better that children should go out, have fun, and feel socially adequate than feel isolated from their peer group. Better to cope with eczema flare-ups in the short term than an isolated child in the long term. Also, the more responsibility children take for their own condition the better. Sooner or later they will decide for themselves the goodies they are prepared to pay the price for and those that are not worth it.

The same principles apply for sleep-overs. If the child is on antihistamines, he or she can still take the dose that will cut down the scratching at bedtime. Obviously the creaming will be curtailed but ensure that your child goes armed with a moisturising cream and, if relevant, a steroid one. If you are worried about other people's bedding, make sure your child takes his own sleeping bag and pillow. And then stop worrying! The more you relax the more relaxed your child will be about his eczema. Above all, encourage your child to be open about the condition. If he or she can say, without embarrassment to friends "This is what eczema is and this is how I treat it" – it's not going to be much of an emotional burden. What's more your child will have a life-gift that is wrapped in gold. The more we can learn to communicate our feelings or problems to others, the less we are trapped by them and the more positive lives we are likely to lead. If your child can do it now with eczema there is no reason why he or she cannot do it with other things forever.

· *Swimming and sport* ·

Encourage your child to join in sporting activities as much as possible. Obviously if the skin is cracked and it is difficult to stretch without cracking the skin still further, the child will have to stay off games until the skin improves. But don't worry too much about the dirt factor in games like football, although, if there are many open or infected sores on your child's legs, he will need to keep them covered or may have to give the sport a miss until the eczema gets better. Sweating can irritate eczema so, if possible, your child should have a shower and change out of sports clothes straight afterwards. Once home, make sure your child soaks in a bath and uses the emollients as described earlier.

Swimming is an activity that can worry parents of children with eczema. It is true that chlorinated water can aggravate the condition and it is not easy to find swimming pools that use an alternative. But swimming is a very important sport for most children, and for a child with eczema who may have a pre-disposition to asthma as well, this activity is very useful in helping develop the lungs. Make sure the child is covered with an emollient cream before entering the water. Keep repeating the message about showering straight after he comes out of the pool. Finally, remember that the skin needs to be moisturised afterwards.

Another issue about swimming which needs to be discussed is the embarrassment factor. With the body so exposed your child may feel embarrassed about his skin condition. He may have noticed stares from other people and felt discriminated against and rejected. If your child is reluctant to go swimming try and find out if this is what is at the back of it. Try and get him to see that he shouldn't be defeated by other people's prejudices and ignorance.

· *Sunlight* ·

Some people find that sunlight improves their eczema while others find that it aggravates the condition. Even if you find that your child's eczema is improved when he is in the sun, you should protect the skin by using a suitable sun-screening product. The higher the SPF (Sun Protection Factor) the more protection is given. Children's skin is very sensitive to the sun and so you should use a cream of SPF 15 or more. If your child is sensitive to colourings and perfumes you will need to avoid products that contain those. Some of the products that seem to suit people with eczema are listed in Chapter 12.

If the skin has been over-exposed to the sun and burning has occurred, bathe in a tepid bath with plenty of bath oils added and apply emollient. After-sun lotions are probably best avoided as many contain antihistamines.

· *Hospitalisation* ·

With the best will in the world and with even the best of parenting, eczema presents a strain on the family. The extra work and worry and tensions of trying to be all things to all people, particularly if there are other children around can become a very heavy burden. So if the doctor suggests that a brief spell in hospital may be a good thing for your eczematous child, don't take it as a failure on your part. Take it as necessary breathing space. Children's eczema does seem to clear up quite miraculously in hospital. Most of us are quite amazed by it if not a little baffled. When the child comes out looking as if he or she has never heard the word 'eczema' we wonder where we are going wrong and feel quite inadequate.

Why does eczema clear up so quickly in hospital when it seems to have taken up permanent hold when the child is at home? A hospital is, to a large extent, a controlled environment which a home is not. There are probably less dust mites, pollens and other eczema-aggravators hanging around hospitals than there are at home.

Maybe the medication gets applied with regularity and precision. Maybe what the child eats is more closely monitored. Who knows? One thing is for certain and that is that children would rather live with eczema at home than without it in a hospital. But a short stay in hospital that will clear up the condition temporarily and give you a break in the meantime is good news. Use it to charge your batteries. Don't camp out in the hospital unless for some reason you have to. Your child will be in a ward with other children and there will be people to look after him and things to play with. Visit, of course, but more importantly, rest and get your strength back.

· *High risk areas* ·

Children with eczema are more vulnerable to catching other people's infections. Usually these present no special problems with the exception of the following two:

● *Cold Sores (herpes simplex)*: These are very contagious and can lead to a very serious, even fatal, viral illness known as *eczema herpeticum*. It is essential that children with eczema avoid all mouth to skin contact with anyone with a cold sore. If your child's eczema suddenly spreads, with a high temperature and infection of the eczema, check immediately with your doctor that it is not eczema herpeticum. If it is, your child will need emergency treatment (see Chapter 11).

● *Impetigo*: this is a contagious, pustular skin disease which can lead to the development of infected eczema.

· *Some children's stories* ·

For Joanna eczema is 'a family thing'. Her story is told by her mother.

· JOANNA ·
(aged seven)

I (Joanna's mother) had severe eczema as a young child. My mother said it started after I had the smallpox jab. My grandmother was so badly affected by eczema she could hardly bend her fingers. Sometimes I couldn't walk as a child. I was unable to bend my limbs. It was crusted and weeping everywhere and where it wasn't weeping there was a rash. I went to school in bandages. They painted me gentian violet once – bright purple all over – and I went to school like that. People wouldn't hold my hands. They all thought it was catching. But I'm not the bullyable type so it never really bothered me very much. But it cleared up when I was about seven, apart from a few minor eruptions.

When Joanna was six weeks she had a rash that looked like eczema to me. The G.P. diagnosed it as such and said that she might be allergic to my milk.

My eczema having become a thing of the past I didn't think about it very much. I was very concerned that the baby should be protected from all the risk elements. I made sure we washed everything in non-biological powder for a month before we had her and so on. I was dedicated to breastfeeding this child because some people had told me that formula milk could trigger it. So she never had a formula feed of any description.

I weaned her totally at 8 months and kept her on Wysoy for about two years. When we took her off Wysoy we put her on sterilised milk. We discovered that initially she could take sterilised milk but she couldn't take pasteurised milk. But then after a while if we boiled the pasteurised milk she could take that.

I was able to give her yoghurt after a while and it didn't make any difference.

We had a holiday in Guernsey recently. I've always got a dilemma with suncreams because she does react to them. It was extremely hot and I used some on her even though she already had some patches of eczema. She was staying with some friends of ours, so I gave them some hydrocortisone to put on her at night before she went to bed. The next morning she was very poorly. I looked at the eczema. It had erupted over most of her body and looked infected. She had a high temperature and was very lethargic. We took her to a doctor immediately, who said that the eczema was infected with the herpeticum virus as well as bacteria. The broken eczematous skin was covered in little white blisters. It was pitiful.

He prescribed Zovirax (an anti-viral ointment) for the Herpes. We had to apply that topically five times a day to every single blister. The child was in agony. She was also given an oral antibiotic and Calpol to bring down her temperature. He said that if the Zovirax didn't have a dramatic effect immediately I should bring her back in the morning. He said: "What it's going to do it will do immediately." I think if it hadn't worked they might have taken her into hospital.

It did have a dramatic effect immediately. The next day she was a lot better. We had to apply the Zovirax (acyclovir) for three days. It scabbed like chicken pox once it started healing. After the three days she was a lot better in herself. She didn't look like a sick child any more, she just looked like a child with eczema.

Joanna doesn't have any problems at school. She's never been bullied or teased. Perhaps some children handle it in a way that stops it happening. Joanna is quite resilient socially.

Joanna absolutely hates the application of the creams. She'd rather itch. But if she's in a really bad state with the itching she comes down crying for the cream and then she's really quite grateful. The surgery here is very good. They have a lot of time for a lot of people. They seem to be genuinely concerned with keeping people healthy. They told me that I was only going there when her eczema was out of control. They taught us how to manage the condition more effectively and how to maintain a healthier skin.

They said: "When it is out of control it's essential to bring it back under control." (We use Betnovate then). "And then every other day, whether or not she has got any eczema visible, you should keep the skin supple with emollients so that it protects itself."

We have been doing this on and off for the past couple of years and it is significantly better when we maintain that regime.

Joanna's quite philosophical in a way. I remember when she was four we were walking to school and she had very itchy eczema on the back of her legs. She kept saying: "I wish I didn't have eczema. I really hate this."

I said: "Cheer up, Joanna, spring's nearly here. It will be better in the warm weather."

She looked up at the sky and smiled and said: "Yes, and summer just comes stealing through the clouds, doesn't it?"

She is always like that. You can reason with her and she lifts herself above it.

Although frightening when it happens, eczema herpeticum is not a rare occurrence and it is not always immediately diagnosed as you will see from Erica's story.

· ERICA ·
(aged 10)

It started when Erica was six months old. She'd always had a dry skin. My brother-in-law had died and during the two days of his burial the eczema came out. Whether she picked up the stress from me I don't know. It was just across her forehead – the weepy pimply type. From then on she was riddled with it all over her body. But she never got it on her face again. It was very itchy, especially at night. She wasn't content until she scratched herself raw and then she would sleep.

She was at her worst during the ages of one to three and then when she was four years old she got eczema herpeticum. It was a Saturday evening. Her hands were blistery and weepy. It was like thousands of taps had been turned on on her hands. We had been in my husband's garage workshop for a few minutes and I thought she might have touched something there, but she said she hadn't. I think you know as a parent when something isn't quite right.

Our G.P.'s surgery was closed and there was a locum on call. I took her out to see him but he made me feel I was wasting his time. He said she had an infection and gave her some antibiotics. Two or three days later she still wasn't getting any better, in fact she was very bad by then. I took her to see my own doctor at the surgery. She was very limp and sleepy so I had to carry her. She had a temperature and was very dehydrated. She was very poorly indeed.

My doctor asked me if anyone in the family had cold sores. I said my husband had. My doctor got straight through to the hospital. She was in there for over a week. For a couple of days she didn't know who I was.

Erica's school life has been very good. When she started there were only 22 pupils in the school. They totally accepted her with her skin. The headmistress has a daughter who had eczema so she's had VIP treatment really. She's always been made to feel normal. I've always encouraged her to do everything. I've tried to take the view that she's got the eczema but the eczema hasn't got her.

For instance swimming obviously dries her out but I don't make a scene about it. I just cream her well when she comes back. If she's needed any creaming at the school they've done it for her.

She did all the sports. She tried to play on it sometimes if she thought she could get away with it. Sometimes if she couldn't catch the ball she'd blame her hands but people ignored her.

Now the eczema's just on her hands. She's still got very dry skin. But apart from that, she's clear.

Here are stories of two young boys with eczema as told by their mothers.

· ORLANDO ·
(aged 8)

Orlando was born with very dry skin but he was all right until he was six months old. Then he developed eczema all over his head. It went after a while and then it appeared behind his ears and his legs. Then it came on his face. The doctors gave him cortisone creams which I wasn't very happy with. His skin never smelt fresh. His body never smelt fresh like a baby's should, because he always had creams on it.

He is a very good child. He is so caring of other people but he is a terrible patient. He hates the creams and he hates all the medicines.

When he was a year old he got asthma as well as the eczema.

I went to see a homoeopath with him when he was about three years old. She was a very nice girl. She gave him these little white pills. One day he was watching me put the pills away. I was busy and when I saw him in the garden, I noticed he was very quiet and I thought he must be up to something. Then I saw he had taken all the pills in one go – the whole bottle! It was a month's supply. I thought: "Is he going to have an asthma attack? Or is his body going to be covered with eczema?" The homoeopath said it wouldn't do any harm. I decided I didn't believe in this stuff any more. One month's supply in one go had no effect whatsoever!

He is a very happy boy. He is clear now except for his fingers, but his skin is dry. He likes the girls, especially the good-looking ones. If the girls look at his hands he gets upset and he says: "Why do I have to have this eczema?"

At one stage, when he was three years old, it was very bad on his eyes. His skin was very sore and it looked like it was going to bleed at any time, it was so thin and fragile. He would lie on the floor and say: "I hardly can see." It was difficult to put cream on because he hated it and would struggle and I felt maybe I hadn't put it on the right place. I took him to the optician to check his eyes out. He decided he was short sighted and sent me to the hospital as well. The doctor at the hospital was horrible to me. The surrounds of Orlando's eyes were so red with eczema that he thought I'd been punching him or something. He said: "Who's done this to him?" I said: "Nobody's done anything to him. It's eczema."

· DUNCAN ·
(aged 6)

Duncan developed atopic eczema at the age of three months. At first it was under control with mild steroid creams, but just after his second birthday, it was as if someone had flicked a switch because suddenly we could not control it. It was all over his body. He only really got it on his face when it was very bad, but the rest of his body was covered. He was a very itchy child.

The next two years were dreadful. We got next to no sleep. We were very tired, worn down and irritable. It was a difficult phase to go through. He used to cry in the night because he would wake up crying and scratching. I would go and join him because my husband couldn't sleep with him scratching if he was in with us. I'd try and leave him if he settled down but I usually ended up back with him.

Our doctor referred us to a local hospital and we visited them on a regular basis. Duncan tried various creams and was even put under a dietitian for a while. We were given a whole load of bandages by the hospital but that was more frustrating for him than ever. He just desperately had to get the bandages off so he'd scratch more.

It was very frustrating not knowing how we could help him.

However, by a stroke of luck, we heard about some trials for evening primrose oil at Charing Cross Hospital. Duncan had tried a course of capsules from our own G.P. but we had not noticed any great improvement. However, these trials involved taking a much higher dose so we decided to give it another go.

We were immediately accepted and right at the very end of the 16-week trial, Duncan's skin started to show signs of improvement. That was just before his fourth birthday and he has continued to take evening primrose oil ever since. His skin has continued to improve to such an extent that for the last year he has hardly suffered from eczema. He now takes eight tablets of 40mg Epogam every day.

5

ECZEMA AT SCHOOL

The best ally your child will have at school is a basic knowledge of the condition. It is virtually impossible to cope with other people's ignorance when you only have a hazy knowledge of the subject yourself. This is true of any age group. It doesn't mean that your son or daughter has to gen up on the pathology of eczema and write a PhD on it. All he or she needs are a few basic facts to counter taunts and prejudices.

· *Talking to the teachers* ·

The second most valuable ally your child can have is an informed and sympathetic teacher. This is where you come in because each year, or whenever the class teacher changes, you will need to go into school and have a little chat about your child and his skin condition. Book an appointment of anything between 15 minutes and half an hour because there is quite a lot to talk about. A child with severe eczema has Special Educational Needs and is entitled to have those needs catered for. So first discuss the basics:

● Explain the condition briefly. It is a hot itchy skin and the desire to scratch may be overwhelming. Telling the child "Don't scratch!" is not going to help, it will only make the child more anxious and the situation worse. Ask the teacher to encourage the child to pat or rub instead of scratching.
● Say that you realise that your child could be disruptive during a frenzied scratching bout, but he is not doing this deliberately, he is in genuine distress. Ask the teacher if he would excuse your child from the classroom to cool down. Explain that your child will probably need to apply an emollient and maybe a cortisone cream to treat the skin. Some schools will allow teachers to do this while others will not. This is discussed in greater detail later on in this chapter.
● Explain that eczema is not contagious. Regardless of what the activity or how close the contact, no one can catch eczema from your child. Tell the teacher that one of the problems is that many people don't know this and may tease or steer clear of your child for fear of catching eczema. If, without making a special case of it, the teacher can explain to all the children that eczema is not catching it

could be beneficial to your child.

● One way the teacher could illustrate this is by personal example. If he or she is seen to give the child a hug or a cuddle (depending on the child's age of course!), it not only gives the green light to others, but helps the child feel less rejected and alienated.

● A child with eczema is more likely to catch other people's skin infections like impetigo, warts, athlete's foot and ringworm as well as cold sores. Ask the teacher to try and avoid contact between your child and one who has *cold sores* (*herpes simplex*) as this could result in your child getting *eczema herpeticum*, a very serious, occasionally fatal, viral illness (see Chapter 11). If your child is in contact with someone who has *impetigo* (see Chapter 11) this could lead to your child's eczema becoming infected. Again contact should be avoided. Very unlikely, but still worth mentioning, is the risk of HIV to your child. There is a slight possibility that this virus can be transmitted through broken skin in eczema, as it can with anyone with breaks or cracks in their skin. So it is important for a person with eczema to avoid coming into contact with the blood or semen of anyone who has HIV. Saliva is not important.

● Help the teacher become aware of some of the problems facing your child at home. Explain that when the eczema is bad your child may have several sleepless nights. He may be suffering the effects of lack of sleep or sedation in class and this may make him inattentive. Also explain that in flare-up situations the child may not be able to attend school for genuine reasons. (But having explained this to the teacher, don't get into a collusive situation with your child and send in sick notes when he could be at school.)

Education is important for everybody. It is particularly important for children with eczema because, as I detail in the next chapter, *Teenagers with Eczema*, there are careers which are difficult if not closed to eczematous people. Many of these are physical or manual and although people with eczema don't have to have a clerical or academic career, they need to get the grades and cover the academic groundwork because the choices are more limited. Added to this is the very real possibility that their education may be disrupted in one way or another: absences from school, inattentiveness because of the itch or antihistamines, difficulty in writing if the hands are affected, difficulty in sitting exams if the conditions are bad and so on. All this can be compounded as the years go by and place your child at a disadvantage if it is not picked up early on.

I'll give you a personal example. Simon's hands were very badly affected when he was first learning to write. There were many times when he could hardly hold a pencil and other periods when he clutched at it awkwardly and with obvious difficulty. Added to this he was absent from school from time to time and when he was there, he was often very tired and sleepy because of endless sleepless nights. This went on for some years. During that time his teachers, although sympathetic to his condition, were obviously reluctant to drive him to form his letters correctly and hold his pencil the right way. They saw this little wizened boy with cracked and weepy hands doing his best. And they probably felt that it was good enough. I can well understand their sentiments.

It wasn't until he was about ten or eleven that we cottoned on to the fact that the undecipherable scrawl that was his handwriting was not going to get better without help. So we took him to a remedial handwriting teacher. Of course at this stage it was very difficult to teach him to re-learn good writing skills because the other had become instinctive. As it was, Simon's writing did get better but he never quite got that easy flow he might have had. If I had picked this up early on I might have been able to put it right.

· *Special educational needs* ·

The 1981 Education Act encourages pupils with Special Educational Needs to attend mainstream schools wherever possible. This doesn't mean that the child is not entitled to special consideration. In most cases teachers will help to create an environment that makes your child's school life easier. You can help them by explaining what those conditions are. Here are some suggestions:

● A cool corner of the classroom, away from radiators, is essential. They should also be seated away from sunny windows.
● A pot of cream, a cool flannel and a cotton sheet can be a lifeline to a hot and itchy child. Also the teacher should encourage the child to leave the classroom for a quiet scratch and to cool down. If this is done with sympathy and without fuss, not only will it not disrupt the class but will help the child to take control of his condition.
● Plastic seats can cause irritation and you can get over this by giving your child a cotton pillow case to place over the chair.
● There are activities which include the use of materials that may aggravate eczema. Play dough, finger paints, sand and water play are examples. It may be that the child can get by with the application of emollient beforehand to act as a barrier, washing well after and re-applying the cream. If this works, well and good; if it doesn't, ask the teacher to find some interesting activity that your child can do in parallel.

For older children glues, paints, clay, chemicals, oils, metals and detergents can pose problems. Protective clothing, emollients, washing or showering after the activity with time given for the re-application of creams may be all that is needed to enable the child to take part. However, in some cases the child will need to be excused a particular activity.

● Cotton mittens or plastic gloves can be useful but should be used only occasionally as over-used can lead to poor finger co-ordination.
● Plastic overalls can be uncomfortable for a child with eczema and elastic at the end of the sleeves can irritate or cut into sore wrists.
● If your child is sensitive to animal fur he may not be able to play with guinea pigs, hamsters or rabbits.
● If your child is sensitive to dust, sitting or playing on a carpet can make the eczema erupt. You can help the school by providing a cotton sheet or pillow.
● Soaps, washing-up liquids and paper towels can all irritate the skin. It is a good idea to provide your child with a soap-substitute, emollient and cotton towel for his own use.
● Explain to the teacher that your child will need somewhere private to apply creams when necessary. Children can be very self-conscious and the last thing a child with eczema needs is to be forced to attend to his skin in public.
● If your child is on a special diet, staff should be made aware of this. If the school provides dinners they may be able to cater for your child's allergies, but you may need to send in fruit juice in place of milk and a substitute pudding. Initially, you will probably need to discuss this with the head teacher.
● As regards sporting activities, explain to the teacher that you would like to encourage your child to take part as fully as possible. However, there are special needs here. First of all chlorine and sweat can both irritate eczema. This can be kept to a minimum if before swimming the child is covered with emollient. He should be given time to shower well after the swim and re-apply the emollient. It may mean that the child has to leave the session a little early to allow for this. With other sports similar principles apply.

You may also need to discuss with the teacher the fact that your child may be reluctant to go swimming or join in sporting activities because of the embarrassment factor. Undressing in front of others if your skin is sore and weepy takes a lot of courage, as does appearing in a bathing costume in that condition. If your child's teachers have not come across severe eczema before, they may not be aware of the psychological implications. You will need to inform them of some of the less obvious aspects of the condition.
● With the previous point in mind, the teachers may well need to look out for teasing and taunting from other children. This is very

difficult to handle without making the child with eczema a special case, which we want to avoid. But if the teachers are aware of the possibility, they may be able to minimise it.

● School uniform can present problems if it is made with an irritant fabric. Cotton is the best next to eczematous skin so you may need to make your own school uniform, although matching the official one may be a problem. You will probably need to discuss this with the head teacher.

The National Eczema Society has produced a special booklet entitled *Eczema in Schools* for teachers and non-teaching staff. You may like to leave it with your child's head teacher. It is available from the NES head office for the price of £2.

· *Legalities* ·

Legally, head teachers do not have to oversee the taking of medicines or the application of creams, but the school's medical officer should note the details of the child's condition in the school records.

In some local education authority areas teachers are specifically not to apply creams or give medicines. If this applies to your area you may have to go into the school once a day to apply the creams. If this is not possible, talk to the head teacher. There may be other parents with eczematous children who would be able to share the responsibility with you.

With older children who can apply the creams themselves, the school staff may be willing to supervise them and check that they are doing it properly. If this is the case, make arrangements to go in and demonstrate the correct procedure so that they know how it should be done.

· *Pilgrims school* ·

According to Bryan Lask, consultant psychiatrist at The Hospital for Sick Children in London's Great Ormond Street, in childhood eczema clinical experience shows that up to 40 percent of patients have some form of psychological problem over and above the skin disorder. Writing in the booklet *Atopic Eczema* for the British Society for Paediatric Dermatology, Mr Lask states:

There is a complex interaction between emotional arousal and eczema. Emotional arousal leads to perspiration and increased sweating, which intensifies the eczema, which in itself becomes upsetting and distressing perpetuating a vicious circle.

Emotional arousal includes everyday situations like anxiety, worry, anger, sadness and feelings of guilt. Add to this the problems the child with eczema may have about his appearance and the teasing and name-calling he may have to put up with on a daily basis, the emotional triggers of eczema are all too obvious.

On top of this, parental attitudes play a strong part with some of us fussing too much and others being too laid back.

When a parent is over-involved and over-protective the child is not encouraged and may not even be allowed to fulfil his potential, [writes Mr Lask]. He is treated as more of an invalid than is necessary and this can reinforce the problem. Parents who deny or play down the severity of the problem do so with the best of intentions, such as the more attention one pays to a problem the worse it will become. This is of course not completely accurate in that frequently urgent attention to exacerbations of the illness is required.

The point is that, as parents, it is hard for us to take a dispassionate view of our children, particularly those with a condition like eczema. Most of us do the best we can, but if a child has become depressed, withdrawn and has missed a lot of schooling, it is probably worth thinking about sending them to a school like Pilgrims which specialises in the care of children with eczema and/or asthma.

The booklet, *Atopic Eczema*, referred to contains papers presented at a symposium on atopic eczema at the Institute of Child Health in 1990. Patrick Murtagh, ex-headmaster of Pilgrims School, says that parents of children with severe eczema often don't get the support they need from society and so need to find specialist help in the shape of his school. Writing in the booklet he says:

To many, asthma and eczema have developed into a crutch, an escape route from difficult or stressful situations and relationships. They lack confidence, are under-achieving and feel like failures, with all that that implies. At Pilgrims we offer a holistic management regime which focuses on the child rather than their medical problem.

This holistic approach includes 24-hour medical cover and regular checking with G.P. and specialists and in some cases regular physiotherapy. Children who have led a sedentary life, or who have shrunken leg tendons caused by walking awkwardly because of the condition, can be helped in this way. The school also encourages a full range of occupational activities to help broaden the children's horizons. But perhaps most beneficial of all, says Mr Murtagh, is the mutual support given by the students to each other.

They can see the changes in each other and know that, with perseverance, they too can benefit if they are prepared to make the effort.

The school fees are paid by the local education authority in which the child lives. It can be a bit of a struggle to get some local authorities to sponsor the child. What needs to be established is that the child has special needs such as 24-hour medication for instance. Parents who are interested in sending their child to Pilgrims would probably be best advised to contact the school initially to find out if their child is a suitable candidate. If so, the school will advise parents on how to approach their local education authority. The stay at the school is usually for a period of two years. During this time children are encouraged to visit home as often as is advisable. Children can come between the ages of nine and 16 (or older than that if there is a special need). The address of Pilgrims School appears in Chapter 17.

Sending a child away is not a concept that comes easily to most parents. We feel guilty; we feel failures; we feel we should be able to cope by ourselves and maybe we also fear the comments of friends and neighbours. Added to this is the feeling that most of us have that we want our children to have normal childhoods and go to ordinary schools. But a child who has had severe eczema for many years, missed a lot of schooling and is feeling isolated and depressed is not experiencing the same childhood as most children. In this situation it is worth looking at Pilgrims School as a possible way of reversing the experience.

According to Mr Murtagh it is not parents who are the most difficult to convince in this respect, but grandparents who, he says, "can be terrors", particularly if the eczema is hereditary. Grandparents, he says, are notorious for saying that they were quite capable of looking after their son or daughter when he or she was a child with eczema so why should it be difficult for the current parents.

I've had grandparents who will not visit their grandchildren unless they could take them away. They cannot stand the idea of leaving them here and they undo all the hard work that the parents have done, [says Mr Murtagh]. The worst case I had was a child who lived with her mother, father, and grandparents and aunty. The first weekend the child was here, she was perfectly all right, but the parents said they had come because they couldn't stand not seeing her. This was breaking all the rules because we ask parents to leave the children alone for the first three weeks to give them a chance to settle in. Anyway, the parents came that weekend. The following weekend the aunty arrived, in floods of tears, saying she couldn't stand being without the child and the third weekend the grandparents came and yanked her away. She was doing perfectly all right. She is now in danger of becoming a permanent invalid.

Diane and Louise are two school children with severe eczema. Both stories are told by their mothers.

· DIANE ·
(not her real name)

The only place Diane hasn't got the eczema is on the palms of her hand and the soles of her feet. The first time I took her to the doctor she was five weeks old. She's 10 now.

On school days she gets up early. She is difficult to wake up because she is tired. She's been up at night. She has her hydrocortisone applied – one for the face and one for the body as well as the very gungey moisturiser which is liquid paraffin. She then has a housecoat on because she can't get dressed. Another reason why she has to get up early is because the creams have to sink in before she can get dressed at all.

She then has breakfast. She is on a restricted diet – preservative, additive and dairy-free. Most meats she can't have. She can only have plain chicken and plain lamb, organic if I can get it. She can only have bottled water and apple juice or herbal tea which she doesn't like. The only cereal she can have is rice because her diet is gluten-free as well.

She'll then dress for school. Normally during the summer term she'll only make a few hours of school. They are unwilling to cream her at school so if that needs doing I have to bring her home. She is paranoid that everyone is looking at her. If she has any problems she thinks it's because of her skin. She's had to put up with name calling. Children will always find something and with Diane it's very easy.

She doesn't cope with the psychological effect at all. She gets very distressed. I have now got through to the school that if she gets very distressed they must ring me. The distress starts off the itching. It's definitely attached emotionally. The second she is in trouble or anxious she starts to scratch.

She's been at the school six years. You have to fight so hard for things that are obvious to us, like sitting her away from sun or heat or dust. She now has a very sympathetic teacher. She will not do P. E. because of what's been said to her in the past by her peer group. I think that could have been stopped. I think in a class of 28 you can see that going on. It would have been a big help. She has a big block now on anything like that.

One incident in particular was when they were working on monkey bars in the gym. All the children were underneath her looking up her legs. That sort of thing happened time after time after time. It was never stopped.

She is now starting to go out a bit more but that development has been very slow. There are lots of things she can't do and won't do. I have to think about it all the time – where she's going, what she's eating and drinking.

Infection is a problem. She was on permanent antibiotics for two years. She's now been taken off those. Occasionally she will have oral steroids which are wonderful. It's like a reprieve. She's in pain a lot and she screams a lot. She objects to the treatment. She gets fed up with it. We can't leave her with anybody or trust anybody to do it in case we regret it later. She has to be cleaned and she has to be creamed. We have tried encouraging her to do it herself but it was not successful.

Most of last year she was bandaged from head to foot. She loathed that. The bandages themselves were an added irritation. She has three-layered bandages when her eczema is bad which she goes to school in quite often. The leg bandages are very hard to keep on. They come off quite often. The kids start on that. I'd take her in and she's in tears and when I'd pick her up she's in tears.

When she has a bad day the whole house has a bad day. We would like to redress that balance. But it is difficult to discipline a child who is suffering herself.

She has a four-year-old sister and a brother who is nearly nine. They don't think there is any room for them to be ill. I have actually not noticed my son for two days when he has been ill. On several occasions when he has had huge blisters he hasn't bothered to tell me. And that is not right. But it takes up so much time and energy and effort – how many pieces can you cut yourself into? I feel my whole life revolve around Diane and they obviously feel that too. They don't feel they are entitled to any of our time.

I actually bathed my son the other night. To feel normal skin is lovely.

Diane can't swim. She's terribly allergic to horses but she insists on riding. She absolutely loves it. It's the only time she is confident. That's her one outlet. Of course horses don't ask questions or make comments.

· LOUISE ·

Louise's eczema started when she was three months old. It abated at five months and did not return until she was 18 months old following three courses of antibiotics prescribed for a chest infection (which in fact was later diagnosed as asthma). Then the eczema

*became chronic and the asthma severe. When Louise was five-and-
a-half the asthma improved but the eczema worsened with a
vengeance.*

*Louise never wanted comforting at the onset of the itch. We had to
let her scratch and then she would come to us for a cuddle. But if we
tried to pick her up at night from the floor where she had crawled to
scratch, she would go into fits of almost uncontainable screaming.
When she had satisfied the scratching urge, which usually took
about 15 to 20 minutes, she would come to us, bloody and shredded,
to be calmed.*

*At school the teachers were supportive but children were children.
She had no friends. She was made to be the last in the dinner queue
and she would walk around with the dinner lady at lunch-time play
because, unknown to us, she was being bullied.*

*Her appearance was horrendous. When she was nine years old
she looked 90. At that time every gland in her body had been
enlarged for about 18 months. The bedding would stick to her. We
had to spread thick cream over her back each morning and use a
wooden spatula to remove thick layers of dried skin. She had a really
tortured existence. It wasn't a childhood. It wasn't a life. I found it
almost impossible to take.*

*We had been trying to get her into Pilgrims School. In fact she had
even been on a visit. Patrick Murtagh, the headmaster, had said to
her: "I am not just saying I think we can help you, Louise, I know we
can." He had given her the world. She had walked around the school
with two girls one of whom had had severe eczema but was now
dancing and going off on an arts course. For Louise it was a glimpse
of what life could be. After all, these were children who had suffered
in a similar way but were now fine.*

*But the wheels are very slow and it took us many months from
when we first enquired to get her into that school.*

*In the meantime she was getting worse and nothing seemed to
help. She'd been referred to a psychiatrist, but he lost credibility
completely when he told her he knew exactly how she felt because
he'd suffered sunburn the previous year. Dermatologists offered
creams which didn't do much and when we rang the hospital in the
middle of the night in desperation they said they would admit her if
they could put her in a psychiatric ward. Well, I wasn't prepared to
go along with that. She needed freedom from pain and she needed to
sleep.*

*We reached the stage where we couldn't get her from the bed.
Louise covered the mirrors because she couldn't bear to see herself.
She wouldn't get up to go to the toilet in case she caught a glimpse of
herself in the mirror there. She screamed if visitors came to the
house because she did not want anyone to see her. She lay in bed
with her sheets up to her nose. But she hardly slept at all. Eventually*

she broke. We'd been through a bad patch with family worries on top of everything else. She lay on the floor and screamed and screamed. She clawed at her throat and tried to pull the ears off her head. For the first time I realised there was nothing I could do. I broke down in front of her.

The doctor came about an hour later. He told me not to worry and that a place would be found for Louise at Pilgrims School immediately. Our local education authority confirmed that a few days later.

The reality of her staying at Pilgrims was very different. She screamed uncontrollably for the first week and she didn't sleep at all from the Monday to the Thursday. The medical officer there was on holiday when she joined the school so he hadn't been able to assess her. However, the matron felt there was something really wrong with this child from the behaviour difficulties that they were experiencing. She took a skin swab. It transpired Louise had two warring bacterial infections and she had had them for several months despite consultant care. So finally she got the right treatment.

When we saw her three weeks later the eczema was clearing. Her whole being looked lighter and she was a different child. She actually smiled. We hadn't had a smile for goodness knows how long. We owe Pilgrims School one life as far as we are concerned. Without that I don't think she would be here now. She would have committed suicide or at best needed long-term psychiatric care.

As it is she has just done her first work experience week on a conservation area. She is 14 years old now. She is brilliant academically with an I Q of 149-plus and in spite of all the schooling she missed as a young child, she is well set to go on to university.

Thirteen-year-old Daniel is an unusual young man, not the least because he feels that most people know and understand about eczema. He believes that it is a pretty common condition and if people haven't experienced it themselves, they must have a near relative who has. His story, which he tells himself, is also interesting because it describes quite clearly how he felt in two of the schools he has attended and the effects each have had on his skin.

· DANIEL ·

I first had eczema as a baby. My mum put some cream on it and it went away. When I was about eight I had to move schools. I was dyslexic and the school I was at didn't have a dyslexia unit which the old one had. I didn't want to move. It meant leaving my twin brother, Simon, and all my friends. I've never been so scared in my life.

The eczema came back in a massive overdose. First of all it was around my mouth which was really painful. We put some vaseline around it which didn't work. Then it came all over my face and body. It was very bad on my hands. My fingers used to be bandaged and sometimes when you removed the bandages there would be nothing but raw flesh.

One morning when I woke up I couldn't move my mouth to speak. I had gone to bed very tired the night before and had forgotten to put the creams on. I thought something seriously wrong had happened to me. I thought they were going to have to do something to my mouth. My mum told me to put my creams on and slowly, over about two hours, it started to ease and I could move it again.

I never really got along in that new school. I didn't like it much and I didn't easily make friends. My eczema stayed bad the whole of the two years I was there. It was the worst time of my eczema. I used to cry I'd get so upset with myself. If it started itching I'd scratch non-stop for about five minutes. I'd stop and if it was still itchy I'd scratch again. And then I'd cry because it was bleeding.

I didn't adapt well to the work: it was different. The way they taught maths, for instance, was different and I couldn't adapt to the new way. It was a pity because I liked maths.

I used to go swimming with the school. I liked swimming a lot but the chlorine affected my skin. It would make it flare up. You have to have a shower afterwards but there was never time. We often finished late and we had three to five minutes to get out. If I didn't properly dry myself I'd be in trouble. Since I only had a certain amount of time to get dried and dressed I wasn't properly dry and then we had a 10-minute walk back to the school. It made my skin sore. Just before we broke up we were seeing how many metres we could do without stopping. I did 2000 metres (about 1¼ miles) which was a lot more than I thought I would do. It took over an hour and my skin was all sore and itchy. But it was worth it!

I now go to Winton (a boy's secondary school in Bournemouth). *It's brilliant. I think it's helped my skin. I've relaxed. I don't get under pressure even when there's stacks of work. When I first went there I wore gloves because of my eczema. Some of the older boys would come up and ask: "Why have you got gloves on?" I'd say: "It's none of your business, but I've got eczema" and they'd walk off. I knew that they knew what it was and it was just a joke.*

I didn't have a bad time with other kids. Most of them understood because it's very common. Most kids get sores or itchiness or something. Everybody seemed to come up to me and say: "I understand." Three-quarters of the boys in my class have either had eczema or had something like it or their sister or mother has got it. They understand it's not your fault.

It's good because it builds up your confidence. You're not

*embarrassed. The school wouldn't allow it. If they knew you were
getting trouble they would sort it out. It's a brilliant system. They
won't allow racism or making fun of people or fighting. If you're not
going to be afraid it builds up your confidence. Ever since my second
year at Winton my eczema has been good. If I'm calm my eczema
doesn't flare up.*

6

TEENAGE ECZEMA

The teenage years can sometimes be the worst for people with eczema. This is not because the condition gets worse at this time: it can get better. As the skin gets greasier the eczema often improves and it is not uncommon for someone who has had eczema severely as a child to become much better at puberty while his non-eczematous friend discovers zits in a big way!

On the other hand, some people find that they have been free of eczema for a while only for it to come back in adolescence: others develop the condition for the first time during the teenage years. It is a very individual condition.

As a child you were very much in your parents' hands when it came to looking after your skin. Maybe they fussed a lot and insisted on creaming you at all times of the day and night. Or perhaps they were very laid back about the whole thing and only got busy when the skin got very bad. However they treated it and whatever you think about the way your parents handled your eczema, the point is that it is becoming *your* responsibility now. Your attitude to your skin is the only one that counts.

The best way to treat eczema is to remember about it at the right times and then do your best to forget about it at other times. Remember you have eczema at bath times and bed times and treat it with the creams as described in Chapter 12. And forget about it when you go out on a date! In other words *take control*. Remember the eczema when you see you have been placed by a sunny window or hot radiator in a classroom and tell the teacher that it will make your skin itch. Get yourself moved to give yourself a chance of forgetting it after that.

Making a fuss is something we all hate and for a teenager the embarrassment is definitely not wanted. But the point is if you get itchy you are going to be noticed scratching anyway, so you might as well get noticed for being a positive person rather than one who gets pushed around.

The basic rule is not to let eczema interfere with your life.

· Treatment ·

Taking control of your eczema is the most important thing you can do for yourself. To do this you need to make a daily routine of bathing in tepid water to which a moisturiser has been added and then apply an emollient afterwards. It is extremely important to keep your skin moisturised and you will need to apply some form of emollient at least two or three times a day. Don't stop doing this as soon as your skin starts looking better as it may not be healed underneath. If you let it get dry it will itch; then you will scratch and you will be back where you started. Keep up the treatment for some time after the skin seems healed and always keep your skin from getting dry. (See Chapter 12.)

If you are using a steroid cream apply it first, before the emollient. Another thing you should do daily is *check your nails*. Make sure they are clean and short. Try hard not to scratch; see if you can get into the habit of patting or rubbing instead.

Also try and avoid the most obvious triggers. Chapter 9 will give you information on all the different environmental factors that can effect your eczema and hopefully you will be able to avoid some of them. Dietary factors are less likely to be a cause of your eczema than if you were very young; and special diets can mean missing out on parties and outings which is the last thing you want to do. On the whole a diet is not the best way to tackle eczema at this time, but if you think something you eat may be triggering the eczema look at Chapters 4 and 9 for ideas. As a rule a balanced and healthy diet that keeps you fit is good for your skin.

· *School or college* ·

Worry and anxiety can aggravate eczema. Emotional upsets which make you perspire can trigger the itching. Everyone at school and college has some worries but you can help yourself by making the environment as comfortable as possible. Check under the heading 'Special Educational Needs' in Chapter 5 and you may find there are things you could avoid.

· *Swimming* ·

Chlorine can aggravate eczema but not usually to the point where you have to give up swimming. You will need to make time to apply the emollients beforehand and shower and re-apply the cream after the swim. Again, try and ignore the hurt and embarrassment. If you notice people staring or looking at you with disapproval just tell them it's not catching and therefore should not concern them.

· *Missing school* ·

Many children miss a good deal of schooling because of eczema. Most of the young people I have spoken to while writing this book have said that much of the time it was not because of the eczema condition but because they couldn't face the teasing of their peer group. Paul, who is now an adult and whose story appears in the next chapter, wrote this description of his school life in *Exchange*, the journal of the National Eczema Society.

> My concern was summoning up the courage to go to school each day to face the same taunts and bullies. The parental advice that I received about these people was that they would soon get fed up with making fun of me and they would then pick on someone else. The truth was that they didn't pick on someone else and they didn't go away: they were there for 13 years.
>
> There is a saying that goes: 'Sticks and stones will break my bones, but names will never hurt me.' In my experience words certainly can brow-beat you into submission, and I have to say that there were times when I deliberately faked illness so that I had a day off from the hassle.
>
> When you've had a particularly bad night and you have slept barely more than a couple of hours; when you've had to get up in the morning to go to school knowing that the first lesson of the day was a chemistry exam; when you know that you aren't going to do well in the test because you've missed the last two weeks' work and you haven't had time to catch up on it; when you feel sore because it is winter time and the bike-ride to school has fairly ripped the skin from your face because it is so cold; and when you then have to face all the name-calling on top, let's just say that it can be very hard putting on a cheery face.

If you are subject to teasing or name calling you can ask your teacher to help. A class discussion during form time on eczema and other conditions could be very valuable. The National Eczema Society has a wide range of literature and posters to help.

If you have missed out on school work, or are going through a bad patch with your eczema, ask for extra work to do at home. Don't leave it to your teachers or parents to suggest it. They may feel bad about putting an extra burden on you. If you feel you can do it, grit your teeth and ask for work! At the end of the day, it is you who will benefit. If you find you cannot understand the work because you have missed the lessons, talk to your teacher and/or your parents. Special coaching, extra lessons or home tutoring may be arranged.

If eczema on the hands makes you a slow worker, try to develop your computer and word-processing skills if you get the opportunity.

Lack of sleep and sleepiness because of antihistamines are common problems for someone with eczema. If you find you are very sleepy in the mornings, try and take the antihistamines earlier on in the evening so that you get less of a hangover effect. Alcohol can increase the sedative effects of a drug like *Piriton* so it is best avoided. Conversely if you find the antihistamine you are on is no longer lessening the itch, it is probably because your body has got used to it. Change to another one.

· *Taking exams* ·

Exam times seem to coincide with high pollen counts and hot weather. This is not good news for a person with eczema, particularly as stress is another aggravating factor. If your eczema is likely to flare up at this time, ask your parents to warn the head teacher in plenty of time so that everyone is prepared should the situation arise. If your eczema is severe the head teacher can inform the examining board who can arrange for you to have extra time to finish each exam particularly if you have, or have had, writing difficulties. They may give permission for you to record answers on tape and they may even re-locate your exams to a hospital ward.

In any event, don't forget to ask your teachers to let you take the exams in a cool room, away from the window. This is not making a fuss – it really does make a difference. And don't forget to wear cool cotton clothes.

· *Careers* ·

It makes sense to take eczema into consideration before embarking on a career as it can flare up again under adverse conditions. Hand eczema in particular can cause problems in certain areas of employment. Here are some of the jobs which may best be avoided:

● *animal handling*: exposure to dander and fur.
● *catering*: constant exposure to water, detergents, raw fruit and vegetables.
● *domestic work*: constant exposure to water, detergents and chemicals.
● *engineering*: constant exposure to cutting oils, suds and lubricants
● *hairdressing*: exposure to water, shampoos and colourants.

● *nursing*: frequent hand-washing, contact with irritants and the risk of cross-infection.
● *The Armed Forces*: entrance requirements, potential exposure to the weather and so on, may cause problems.
● *Work with cement*: because of the chromate in cement.

You can see why a good, all-round education is so important! Jobs that require a good deal of exercise in the brain department are not at all harmful to the person with eczema!

· *Adult eczema* ·

As a teenager you should read the next chapter as most of the information given there is very relevant to you.

· *Teenagers' personal stories* ·

Here are personal accounts from three teenagers who have had eczema most of their lives.

· SHELLEY ·

I've had eczema since I was a baby. It was reasonably bad when I was little; then it cleared up but when I was 15 I got some kind of a blood virus. And then the eczema really flared up. It started gradually and then all of a sudden it was everywhere: all over my body; all my limbs; my trunk and my face. It was raw most of the time.

I was so itchy all the time I was nearly out of my mind. I couldn't stop myself scratching but I got very scared when I scratched because I knew what the result was going to be. I just couldn't stop myself. I used to rip my skin open.

I couldn't sleep. I'd snatch about 10 minutes here and there. I couldn't lay the quilt over me. It hurt to lie down on the bed. As soon as I had contact with the sheet it would aggravate the eczema or the sheet would stick to my skin.

I tried to have a bath as often as I could to keep down the infection but it was very, very painful. My mum used to bathe me which was embarrassing because of my age. I needed to have baths regularly but it was so painful I would cry. I had the emollient creams and steroid creams as well as antibiotic tablets. It would calm it down for a few days but it would just erupt again. Nothing seemed to help at all.

Because it was all over my face people would stare at me. One woman was walking along staring at me and she actually knocked into my mum because she wasn't looking where she was going. It's funny now but at the time it really upset me. I just burst out crying. Sometimes when I went shopping the sales assistants would drop the money on the counter because they weren't watching what they were doing, they were watching my face. It was very upsetting. In the end I never went out of the house. I didn't even like members of my family coming around – just my mum and dad and that was it.

Looking back on it now I don't know how I coped. I couldn't walk because of the eczema and I couldn't put my clothes on because I was too sore. I just sat in the house with a pair of knickers on. Because it was so raw I was hot all the time. It felt as if I was on fire. Even in the middle of winter I had to have fans going all over the house.

I was sent to the skin clinic at the hospital and they did patch tests on me. But the only thing they found I was allergic to was plaster! They tried to help but my skin was no better and eventually they said to me, "There's nothing more we can do for you, Shelley, don't come back unless it gets worse." As I felt at the time that it couldn't get any worse, I was not happy with that at all, but there was nothing I could do.

My emotions were in a complete turmoil. I would continually cry and become very depressed. Other times I was very angry and often asked myself the well-known cliché "Why me?" I would long for a cuddle from my mum and dad, but this wasn't possible as it was just too painful. Other times I would feel immense guilt for what I felt I was putting my mum and dad through. My mum looked after me 24 hours a day. They would take it in turns to stay up all night with me; then dad would do a full day at work. I became their focus in life which I felt very guilty about, but I couldn't cope without them.

Eczema doesn't just affect and take control of the sufferer, but those who care too.

We tried a homoeopath – again it got better for a little while, a few days, and then it just erupted again and sometimes got twice as bad. My mum was at her wits' end. She phoned the National Eczema Society and they recommended going to see Dr Rustin in London, which I did.

First of all he put me on lots of steroids to take orally. It was quite a high dose – six a day for about a month. My skin had to be completely clear before I was put on the Chinese herbal tea. After taking the steroids and before taking the tea I had to take four packets of Chinese herbal granules a day in order to see if I was suited to the treatment, which I was.

My skin cleared completely and I started taking the tea. The eczema started to come back in a few patches but it was found that I wasn't on the right dose. I was taking less than I should. The dose was put up to four tea bags. Again it started to come back all over my body but it was just dry patches. The only rawness was on my arms. I'm now on six tea bags and it has completely gone again except for one patch on my arm which doesn't seem to go at all. Apart from that it is absolutely brilliant. It's all gone off my face which makes life easier to cope with.

The tea is disgusting to taste – really foul! It's two full cups which you have to drink within an hour of brewing. It's quite thick and very strong. My dad says it looks a lot like Camp coffee.

I still have oilated baths and use emollient creams regularly. I don't eat dairy products or a lot of flavourings and colourings.

Shelley's skin has been clear now for about nine months. She has been able to resume her studies at college.

· CHLOE ·
(not her real name)

I had severe eczema as a baby. I was born with very dry skin. When I was about six or seven I was in hospital. I was in there for a month. It was very bad then. It was on my arms, my elbows, legs, and face. My body was okay. It was hard when I was little. My hands were very disfigured and the skin was cracked. I got teased a lot. Kids didn't want to share books with me. I used to cry going to school. I used to hate it. No one wanted hold my hand and they'd say: "Ugh, I'm not touching her" and that sort of thing. After I made some friends it was all right. They were all right with me because they knew me.

After I came out of hospital when I was seven it was loads better. I was fine until I started secondary school. About half-way through the second year it really started to come up. We thought it was something to do with the fact that the school changed sites. We had a new school. As soon as I went there it came up but we never managed to narrow it down to anything. I became very self-conscious about it and I missed a lot of school and I was in hospital again. I was off three days a week sometimes.

I found it difficult to handle socially. When it got bad I was very self-conscious about it. I still am. I use a lot of strong steroids. I am looking for alternatives now, because I am using a lot of steroids on my face especially. It's going to have a detrimental effect after a bit.

A lot of the time I miss school is because I am so self-conscious about it. And I get very depressed. It's still on my face. At the moment it's good but that's only because of the steroids. My mum said: "No more steroids. I am not going to let you use any more steroids – you're just wrecking your face."

I'm on antihistamines at night and a reduced dose during the day. The reduced dose doesn't work that well. A lot of the time when the skin came up, I'd take Phenergan and I'd have to go home because Phenergan really makes me sleepy. I used to get very itchy in class. Now I don't, because of the steroids.

It used to make a difference where I sat in the class. I used to prefer to sit in the middle because I get hot in the summer if there are windows all round. At school you can get quite hot and that's sometimes hard. The teachers have been really good.

I got very behind with my school work. When you're having three days out of school it's hard to catch up. You can copy up from friends' work but you don't have the understanding there or anything. In exams I get very tense and that brings the skin up. This year I've started my GCSE course work and I've pulled my socks up. I've realised that I've got to get on with it, but it's very difficult.

· DANIELLE ·

I've had eczema since I was born. It fluctuates, appearing on different parts of my body at different times. It seems to come when I'm stressed or when I'm hot.

I got it really badly just recently on my hands. It only used to be on a couple of my fingers but it spread. It came on both my hands, my palms and on the sides of my hands. It was a mess. That was in February and I was due to sit my A Levels in June.

It was really horrible to write because it was difficult to rest my hand on the page. There was also a patch where I hold my pen. It was infected and puffy and weepy. It was really painful to write and I would have to bandage my hand up. It was like that for about a week.

I put a strong steroid cream on it which was also anti-bacterial and it got better. But it never went away completely. I am really bad at using the creams every day so it comes and goes.

It was bad while I was still at school because I think we were all 'hyping' each other up about the exams. But when it came to the Easter holidays it died down because I was at home on my own revising most of the time. During the exams I didn't see anybody and it died down then. I used the cream a lot at that time.

It makes my hands really sore to do things. It's a really greasy cream I use for my hands, so when I put it on I can't touch anything. I have to sit there with my hands out in front of me not doing anything. It's a pain.

I sometimes get quite embarrassed when I have to hold my hand out for change. People look at my hands and ask: "What have you done to them? Have you burnt them or something?"

Incidentally, Danielle did very well in her A levels achieving one A and two B grades.

7

ADULTS WHO HAVE ECZEMA

One in eight children have eczema at one time or another as do one in twelve adults. Some of the latter are adults whose eczema has lingered on, while others will have eczema for the first time in adulthood. Some people will have had eczema for the first time as babies or young children and then experience several years of remission only to have the eczema re-appear suddenly and sometimes severely in their adult years.

Since one of the homilies that seems to have attached itself to the condition is "you will grow out of it", it is small wonder that adults with eczema often become quite desperate, believing that they are stuck with it for life. This is not necessarily the case. Adult eczema often does recover completely.

· *Stress* ·

As people get older emotional stress and tension can play a large role in triggering a flare-up of eczema or aggravating the current condition. No one can get rid of stress in their lives, but we can learn how to handle it.

Our bodies are not really equipped to cope with long periods of stress. Centuries ago when we were hunters the body was tuned to quick-action stress. When faced with a threatening situation we either stood our ground and fought or ran. This fight-or-flight response has become part of our psychological and physical make up.

When we prepare for action the brain receives a warning signal. This triggers a chain reaction throughout the body. The adrenal glands secrete *adrenalin* and this mobilises the body's defences, preparing it to fight or run. The heart pumps more blood and more oxygen to the muscles. Blood vessels in the skin and stomach constrict to allow more blood to be diverted to the brain. The lungs bring in more oxygen. The body temperature rises and we start to sweat in order to cool down. At this point another hormone, *cortisol*, is released by the adrenal glands in order to gather energy from other parts of the body to stabilise the situation.

This was all very well for primitive man but it does not do much in helping us cope with the kind of stress we are faced with today.

People often think that stress accompanies a person who leads a very busy life, taking on more than he or she can possible do. Yet many people with eczema restrict their lives because they don't want to be seen in public when their skin looks too awful. Staying at home, feeling bad about yourself, is a very stressful thing to do. While eczema should never be ignored or neglected, it is not a good idea to focus on it heavily either. It is embarrassing to be stared at, but better that than become a self-made prisoner.

Paul, whose story appears later on in this chapter, used to go to school looking like, as he says, 'Michelin Man', he was so heavily bandaged. Today he spends much of his time as a naturist. His eczema still exists and is at times still severe. You do have to adopt a bit of a 'me first' attitude and do what you enjoy.

It may be that all you need is a practical way of handling a build-up of stress. Do you make time for yourself, or are you at everybody else's beck and call? Relax by making time to do something that you enjoy, regularly. This can be a hobby, sporting activity or anything else that you like, so long as you do it often enough.

· *Practical steps* ·

The first step is to get a medical diagnosis of the condition. There are several different types of eczema which share some of the same symptoms like rough scaling, soreness, red spots, dryness, blisters which burst and weep, and constant irritation. Although symptoms may be similar and routine management likewise, there are special treatments that specific skin conditions respond to which your doctor could prescribe. (See Chapter 11 for the most common types of eczema. Atopic eczema is the subject of the major part of this book.)

· *Treatment* ·

The byword with eczema treatment is to act promptly. If it suddenly flares up, don't ignore it. Remember that eczema can become infected. This still does not mean that it becomes infectious: eczema is *never* infectious.

If the eczema is an on-going condition, get into a daily routine of bathing in tepid water which has had an emollient added to it. Apply a moisturiser at least twice twice a day and if you are using steroid creams, remember to apply them before moisturiser (see Chapter 12).

Signs of infected eczema are a deterioration in the condition together with weeping and crusting, yellow pus spots and swollen glands. Please go to your doctor if this happens as you will need special creams and maybe oral antibiotics to treat it. (See Chapter 11.)

· *Keeping eczema at bay* ·

There are a number of ways in which you can cut down the possibility of triggering or aggravating the eczema (see Chapter 9). Here is a quick checklist:

● Wear cotton next to your skin. Synthetic or woollen clothes and bedding can cause over-heating. Some people can get away with putting woollens over cotton clothes.
● Use soap-substitutes and mild shampoos.
● People with atopic eczema may be allergic to dust, dust mites, grass seeds, pollens, feathers and animal fur and dander.
● Use non-biological soap powders and detergents.
● Use cotton mitts at night to stop you scratching and take antihistamines to curtail the itchiness and to help you sleep.
● Dietary factors are not commonly associated with adult atopic eczema so do not embark on a diet without consultation with your doctor or dietitian. Food additives are the most likely to cause problems, particularly artificial colourings and preservatives (see the next section).
● Over-heating, frosty weather, low humidity, dry air, central heating, air conditioning and car heaters can all aggravate a dry skin and eczema.
● Get to know your own triggers. What sparks off one person's eczema doesn't necessarily trigger another's.

· *Diet* ·

Allergic reactions to food are rare with adults with atopic eczema. Eggs can be a problem for some people but it is rare and allergy to milk is even less likely. Along with colourings and preservatives, salicylates may cause problems. These appear widely in our diet, particularly in citrus fruits and apples. They are also included in aspirin tablets. Reactions to additives and salicylates do not seem to be a true allergic response and at present there are no tests available to identify them.

However, you can try and identify adverse reactions to foods by keeping a diary for at least a couple of months. Write down everything you eat and also note the state of your eczema. You may be able to relate the two. A diary may also give you an indication of any excessive amounts of foods that you are consuming. If it turns out that you drink a lot of artificially coloured drinks or eat a lot of heavily preserved and flavoured food, you could well find that switching to a more healthy diet with naturally flavoured wholefoods, could make a difference to your skin condition.

If this is not the case you could try a simple exclusion programme. The first thing to exclude is artificial colourings and preservatives as well as the culprit E numbers mentioned in Chapter 4. If you are heavy imbiber of apple or orange juice, omit those too. In addition exclude any foods that you suspect may be triggering your eczema. Do this for a month to clear the system. If the eczema is no better, abandon the diet. If it improves, re-introduce the abandoned foods to your diet one at a time, leaving a week before each new food. If the eczema gets worse, exclude that food again. If the condition stays the same, bring the food back into your diet.

If you are excluding a number of foods, particularly in an ongoing diet *you must seek the advice of your doctor or specialist*. It is very important for your physical health and well-being to have a balanced diet. Calcium is very important for adults to ensure healthy bones and so are vitamins and minerals. Rigid dieting can be harmful because, if diets are not well balanced, they can be nutritionally inadequate. Furthermore, rigid dieting can involve a very restrictive life-style which can be very stressful and aggravate the eczema.

Dietary treatment in adults has a very minor part to play in the treatment of atopic eczema. Looking into environmental causes is a much more effective line of action.

· *Eczema at work* ·

Allergic contact dermatitis and *irritant contact dermatitis* are two forms of eczema which can be triggered or exacerbated at work (see Chapter 11). Some jobs are particularly hazardous because they are likely to aggravate the condition and can also cause eczema which has been in remission to flare up again. The jobs in this category are catering, engineering, hairdressing, animal handling, domestic work, nursing, work with cement and the armed forces (see Chapter 6).

It is sometimes possible to reduce the risks by wearing barrier creams and protective clothing. If you are having skin problems and you think it may be triggered by something at work, it is worth checking it out with a dermatologist to try and identify what the culprit is.

· *Social and sexual problems* ·

One of the main problems of eczema socially is that there are still many members of the population who think it may be contagious, infectious or unhygienic. Many people with eczema on their hands get embarrassed because they see people staring at them. If you can't say it outright, try and slip into the conversation that you have eczema and that it is neither infectious nor contagious and certainly not unhygienic. You may like to make a joke about how often you have to bathe and how scrupulous you have to be with your laundry and house cleaning. A joke that's not really joke is a very powerful way of getting a message across! If you have eczema on your hands you may find wearing cotton mittens helpful in this respect.

Don't stay away from life or wait until your eczema disappears before you enter it. Friendships are very important to all of us and the person with eczema is no different. You don't have to be the life and soul of the party or go to parties at all if you don't like them. Better to find interests and activities that you enjoy and try and forget about the eczema. This way you can meet kindred spirits, most of whom will be far more interested in you than in your skin condition.

Within a sexual partnership eczema can cause physical problems which then go on to have an emotional effect. If the skin is hot, itchy and sore the person may not be able to bear being touched. The genital area may be affected. Eczema in this area can be severe, making intercourse painful if not out of the question. There are many possible triggers:

● Vaginal deodorants
● Contraceptives including rubber sheaths, caps and spermicidal jellies and creams.
● Sanitary towels and tampons.
● Talcum powder, perfumed soaps and bubble bath.
● Nylon underwear. (Stick to cotton.)
● Very tight clothing and clothing that rubs.
● Rough toilet paper.

Don't try and treat it yourself and don't put steroids on this sensitive area of your body. It may not be eczema that you have. It may be thrush (candida) which requires different treatment. So go to the doctor and get the condition both diagnosed and treated.

If the condition is in the genital area you may have to accept that for a period you may not be able to have sexual intercourse. But this does not mean that you cannot have a sexual relationship. If the woman has the condition she can lie with her partner and caress him to orgasm. It may be that the touching may not be able to be reciprocal but at least the sexual door is not closed. Equally, if the man has eczema and cannot have penetrative sex, he too can pleasure his partner and be pleasured by her without penetration taking place. This is very similar to the sexual enjoyment that many couples give each other after the birth of a baby when sex is also limited.

The most important aspect is to literally keep in touch and to be affectionate to each other. People with eczema need to feel loved and not rejected. But equally, they need to recognise that the condition can make them irritable and this is communicated to the partner who may not always shrug it off or put it down to the condition and may, instead, feel rejected themselves. In many ways it is up to the partner with eczema to take the sexual initiative. You know what you can do and what you can't do as well as what hurts and what doesn't. Your partner may be nervous of approaching you because he or she does not want to give you any more physical pain than you have already. Equally, he or she may feel the approach will be met with rejection and you don't have to have eczema to fear that.

Kissing, cuddling and holding hands are all loving gestures which make the other person feel wanted and desired. Obviously if the whole body is affected, it could become a very isolating experience – for both the person with eczema and his or her partner. Try and stay in touch on an emotional and feeling level. Talk about how you feel and listen in to your partner's feelings. In the same way as you reverse the dry skin situation with the regular application of creams, reverse the isolation experience by getting to know the people who love and care about you.

Try and separate the person from the condition. You are a person: your partner is a person. Eczema is a condition so that is the odd one out. With any chronic condition the person with the illness and the illness itself get locked into a relationship and everyone else is kept outside. Eczema can take over your body and make you feel hot, itchy, sore, tired, irritable, dirty, unlovable and unloved. Well, the condition may be *on* your body, but don't give it house room in your mind. Stay connected to the outside world and particularly to your loved ones.

If you are finding it hard to cope with your emotional life and your love life, it might be worth going to see a counsellor. *Relate counsellors* are well trained and regularly assessed. Furthermore, in most branches there are sex therapists who are also trained counsellors. You can find the address of your local *Relate* branch in the area telephone book.

Alternatively you may like to try and treat the eczema in this part of your body through hypnotherapy (see Chapter 14).

· *Pregnancy* ·

Since eczema is such an individual illness, it varies from person to person as to when it will flare up and when it will remit. A study reported in the British Journal of Dermatology in 1991 found that 52 percent of women experienced an adverse effect on their eczema during pregnancy, usually starting in the first 20 weeks. For 24 percent of women in this study the eczema improved during pregnancy. It was a small study and may not be representative of the population as a whole.

Some people suddenly develop eczema during pregnancy. Others find it flares up then while the more fortunate experience remission during this time. At present whys and wherefores are not known except for the fact that an upheaval of hormones makes a difference to the skin. What we do know is that you need to be careful with treatment during this time. So please keep in regular contact with your doctor.

Topical steroids are generally considered to be safe in eczema treatment provided they are used in limited quantities and under a doctor's supervision. Studies on animals have shown that *topical corticosteroids* on pregnant animals can cause abnormalities to foetal development. These include cleft palate and intra-uterine growth retardation. There is a very small risk of similar effects on the human foetus.

If you possibly can, try and stick to emollients and bandaging to treat the condition. Bandages impregnated with ichthammol or coal tar pastes can be helpful. *Phenergan,* which has a long record of safety, may also be prescribed to help counteract the itchiness.

Obviously herbal remedies like Chinese medicine are not allowed during pregnancy, but you could try relaxation and meditation techniques to try and cope with the stress.

Investigate environmental triggers, such as the ones listed earlier on in the chapter and in Chapter 9, to try and combat the condition at this time.

Diet should never be contemplated without the guidance of a dietitian during pregnancy.

Some mothers with a history of atopy in the family or who already have an eczematous child, may wonder if they should avoid common dietary triggers like eggs and cow's milk during pregnancy. There is some evidence that some babies may become sensitised to these products before birth and this may take place in the womb. But there are no conclusive findings at present. Please don't embark on any diets cutting out these important foods without qualified and expert medical help. A healthy diet with plenty of essential vitamins and minerals and a minimum of junk food is good news for any foetus and a good start in life for any baby.

· *Will your child have eczema?* ·

The predisposition to eczema is an extended family situation. Even if neither parents have the condition, but a grandparent, aunt, cousin or nephew have one of the atopic conditions, there is a possibility that a child of that family will get eczema. Atopy affects one in three people. That puts a lot of people in the target area.

But what is the situation if you, as a parent, have one of the atopic diseases (eczema, asthma or hayfever)? In his book, *Your Child with Eczema*, Dr David Atherton explains:

> If one parent has or has had one of these conditions, the child's risk of developing atopic eczema will be about double that of a child whose parents have never had any of these. If both parents have or have had any atopic disease, the risk of eczema in their child is doubled again. Having a brother or sister as well as one parent with atopic disease does not appear to increase the risk any further. If parents, or brothers or sisters have a history of eczema itself, rather than just asthma or hayfever, then the risk is increased even further.

But bear in mind something else: you don't inherit eczema, you inherit a predisposition to it. Whether the eczema actually develops and whether or not it appears in a mild or severe form is thought to be determined as much by environmental factors as inheritance. A parent with eczema who knows about triggers in the shape of dust mites, pets, pollens, laundry products, foodstuffs and so on is going to be well equipped to help keep the condition buried in the genes rather than running riot on the skin. An eczematous parent who knows about routine treatment and understands the psychological issues involved with eczema, should it appear, is far more likely to be able to keep it under control than someone for whom the condition appears in shock-horror form out of the blue.

· *Cosmetics* ·

Cosmetics can make a big difference to how you look and go a long way to boost your confidence. However, people with eczema do have to be careful about what they use on their skins as they can have allergic reactions to some of the ingredients.

Perfumes and preservatives are two common allergens and some eczema people are allergic to lanolin.

Perfume

Many different ingredients are included to create a perfume and each of these constituents can cause an allergic reaction. Allergy is seldom confined to a single brand of perfume. You may need to avoid any product containing perfume. Some people with eczema can tolerate perfume if it is dabbed on their clothing but others cannot.

Obviously if you are sensitive to perfumes it is best to go for products that do not include them. Hypoallergenic products do not include perfume and although with these products the risk of allergy and sensitivity is reduced, it is not removed altogether.

Preservatives

Preservatives are used to stop products 'going off'. Some products include more than one preservative.

If you are using a product that is preservative-free check carefully the sell-by date (if provided) as bacterial and fungal contamination will start within days or weeks of opening. Also some of these products contain alcohol which limits the growth of bacteria but is not good for eczematous skin because it is drying.

Labelling

There is no legal requirement at present to provide product information. Sometimes manufacturers choose to include only an incomplete list of ingredients or no information at all. Listed below are manufacturers who provide full ingredient labelling. In so doing they provide a real service to people who need to have this information.

- Shisedo
- Potter & Moore
- Christy
- Cover Girl
- RoC

Some products that are labelled 'natural', 'organic' or 'herbal' may not be suitable for eczematous skin as they may contain common allergens. Organic ingredients can produce sensitivity and these products may include preservatives and perfume unless they say otherwise. 'Natural' does not mean safe.

Patch testing

If you don't know the ingredients of a cosmetic or have never tried it before, a good way to find out whether or not it agrees with you is by means of a home patch test (not to be confused with the clinical patch testing that is explained in Chapter 13). Test it on a two-inch square of skin on the upper outer arm for several days. Most manufacturers now provide samples or allow the assistant to test some on you. Explain to the assistant that you have a sensitive skin and you need to try before you buy. Always try this test on any product that you have been using but is now being sold in a 'new and improved' version. It may not be an improvement for you! Sometimes the reaction to a patch test can be very strong, so use tiny amounts and don't do it the day before you have an important engagement.

If you do react to a cosmetic it may be worth finding out what the ingredient is that is causing the trouble. Ask your G.P. to refer you to your local dermatologist for allergy testing. Keep the product that seems to have caused the problem. When the dermatologist has identified the ingredient that is causing the allergy you can write to the manufacturer for advice on their products. Alternatively, you can contact the Cosmetic, Toiletry and Perfumery Association, 35 Dover Street, London W1X 3RA, giving details of the ingredient(s) that are causing the allergy and they will put you in touch with companies that are involved in their dermatology scheme whom you can write to to get specific help.

Cleansing and moisturising

Cleansers work by absorbing grease, dirt and make-up. A gentle cleanser or cleansing bar may work well for your skin. Avoid soap as it dries the skin. A soap-substitute is a much better choice. If you want to tone the skin after cleansing, choose a toner that is alcohol-free.

Emollients are a very important part of good skin care for anyone with eczema, or you may prefer to try moisturisers. If in doubt about their suitability, try the patch test.

Lanolin, which is a fat derived from sheep's wool, is used in many cosmetics because of its moisturising properties. Some people with eczema are allergic to it. If you are, avoid all products that contain lanolin or wool alcohol.

General toiletries

Deodorants and antiperspirants cannot be tolerated by many people with eczema. Many antiperspirants contain alcohol and perfume and can cause an irritant reaction.

Many people with eczema also cannot use talcum powder as it is often highly perfumed and is quite drying to the skin.

Hair removal products are not very well tolerated by people with eczema. Hot wax treatments are unsuitable because eczematous skin is very easily irritated. Bleaching is not recommended and hair removal creams often cause irritation. The best method is dry shaving, or, if you prefer, a wet shave using a soap-substitute, and apply emollient afterwards.

Make-up

Foundation creams can present a problem to some people with eczema. Irritation is more likely to be the problem than allergy: some also contain sunscreens which you may find you are sensitive to.

Lipsticks often contain lanolin, perfume and antioxidants all of which may cause problems.

The dyes in eye make-up don't usually cause irritation or allergy, but the brushes or pads to apply them may give you a problem.

Nail varnish and enamel are usually no problem on the fingers themselves but they can affect any area of skin they come into contact with, particularly any part of your body that has eczema which you scratch.

Camouflage

You may like to try camouflage make-up if the eczema persists or where there is flushed skin or broken veins. Almay, Avon, Clinique, Max Factor and RoC make camouflage creams. Some of these are waterproof which is useful if you are swimming; some include sunscreen. They are available in a wide variety of skin tones and can be used by men, women and children of all races. Other camouflage creams are Veil, Covermark, Keromask and Boots Covering Cream.

Alternatively, the Red Cross offers a service for people with severe eczema who would like to learn camouflage techniques. You can have a session lasting approximately one hour in which you have your skin colour matched with the camouflage creams. These have been specially formulated and have a very high pigmentation – something like six or seven times the pigmentation that you get in ordinary make-up, and hence a lot of covering power. You also discover which creams work best for you. Clients are also shown how to apply the creams and how to make them waterproof so that you can swim with them on.

The Red Cross say that to get a good result it is best to work on a stable surface and in this respect the eczematous skin, with its flakiness, can provide some problems. But if the condition has stabilised or if the problem is scarring, the camouflage process can work quite well. Before receiving this service you have to be referred by your doctor, dermatologist or consultant to ensure that it is suitable and safe to apply the creams.

The consultation is free but contributions are welcome. If you want to know more about this service get in touch with your local Red Cross branch headquarters and ask to speak to the Therapeutic Beauty Care Officer.

· *Shaving (for men)* ·

It is best to avoid shaving foam, astringents and after-shave as they usually contain perfume and sometimes alcohol and can aggravate the eczema. Dry shaving is usually the best, and you should always apply emollient after shaving. If you prefer to wet shave use aqueous cream, a soft emollient cream or bath oil in place of soap or shaving foam.

· *Hairdressing* ·

Many hair products can produce allergic reactions, particularly permanent dyes which can even affect people who have been dyeing their hair for many years. The contact dermatitis which follows produces itching and weeping of the forehead, neck and behind the ears. Where there is a severe reaction, not only is the entire face involved but the problem can spread to the shoulders and the rest of the body. It is very important to follow the manufacturer's advice to dab-test before using any permanent dye. If you have had an allergic reaction with a dye, never use it again.

Perfumes and preservatives are usually included in gels, mousses, sprays, conditioners and so on and these can produce allergic reactions on the face, scalp, neck and ears. If you are using any of these products protect the hands with gloves. You can use the thin disposable polythene gloves or the protective PVC ones with cotton inners.

To be absolutely safe avoid perming, straightening, bleaching, dyeing, hot-brushing, heated rollers, curling tongs and hot-oil treatments.

· *Swimming and sunbathing* ·

Chlorine can irritate the eczema, but so long as you apply an emollient before you enter the water to act as a barrier, remember to shower as soon as you come out and re-apply the emollient or another moisturisers to stop the skin becoming dry, the enjoyment of swimming should more than compensate for some of the more negative aspects.

As for sunbathing, you may find that sunlight improves the condition or you could find that it makes it worse. Obviously if the sun makes the eczema worse you will stay out of it, but even if it improves the skin, you must protect it from over-exposure to ultraviolet rays.

● Remember exposure to the harmful rays of the sun is greatest when the sun is high in the sky, between 11 a.m. and 3 p.m. Try and limit the amount of time you spend out of doors at this time and, if you are out, stay in the shade as much as possible.
● Loose, long-sleeved cotton tops and trousers will protect you from the harmful rays as will a sun hat (particularly if it has a wide brim).
● Always use a sunscreen. The higher the SPF (Sun Protection Factor) the more protection is given. If your skin burns easily you should use a product with an SPF factor of 15 or more. People with darker skin that tans easily and rarely burns can usually get away with an SPF factor of around 10.

If your eczema gets worse in sunlight use a cream of SPF 15 or more, regardless of your skin type. You should re-apply the sunscreen every two hours. If you are swimming choose a water-resistant one, but still re-apply frequently.

Sunburn is due, in the main, to ultraviolet rays and these penetrate into water and are also reflected off sand. Radiation mostly comes from the blue sky and not from the sun so even if you are sitting under a parasol, you could be vulnerable.

Products that seem to suit people with eczema are listed in Chapter 12.

If the skin has been over-exposed to the sun and burning has occurred, bathe in a tepid bath with plenty of bath oils added and apply emollient. After-sun lotions are probably best avoided as many contain antihistamines and may cause an allergic reaction.

· *High risk factors* ·

People with eczema are more vulnerable to catching other people's skin infections. Usually these present no special problems with the exception of the following three:

● *Cold Sores (herpes simplex)*: These are very contagious and can lead to a very serious, even fatal, viral illness known as *eczema herpeticum*. It is essential that you avoid all mouth-to-skin contact with anyone with a cold sore. If you fancy someone and they have a cold sore, please wait until it goes before you get physically involved. Also be careful about sharing cups that haven't been washed, and so on. You do really need to be scrupulously hygienic under these circumstances.

If your eczema suddenly spreads, is infected and you have a temperature, check immediately with your doctor that it is not eczema herpeticum (see Chapter 11).

● *Impetigo*: this is a contagious, pustular skin disease which can lead to the development of infected eczema.

● *HIV (the AIDS virus):* This virus can be transmitted through eczema and broken skin. The known risks for acquiring HIV are by unprotected penetrative sexual contact (vaginal or anal intercourse) with an infected person. You can also become infected through sharing blood-contaminated equipment (needles, syringes and so on) with an infected person, or transfusion of unscreened infected blood or blood products. The virus can also spread from an infected mother to the foetus or newborn infant across the placenta, during delivery or by breast milk.

Body fluids that carry significant amounts of HIV with a potential for transmission are blood, semen, female genital secretions and breast milk. Saliva, urine, faeces, sweat, vomit and nasal secretions do not present significant risk unless they are visibly contaminated with blood.

Normally skin is a very good defence against HIV and other infective agents. But people with active, weeping eczema or eczema with skin cracks should either avoid contact with HIV-infected body fluids or ensure that additional protection is present where contact with HIV-infected body fluids is likely.

The main part of the body at risk will be the hands, so latex gloves would provide a suitable barrier in situations where contact is likely (for example, during contact with bleeding sites on potentially infected persons, or during mutual masturbation). Small areas could be covered with plastic-type dressings for the duration of contact. Infected persons should use a condom to reduce further any exposure to semen or genital secretions.

If you are uncertain what to do or what level of risk applies, you should discuss the matter with your doctor. Health care workers with extensive active eczema should seek professional guidance on possible re-allocation to duties not involving patient contact until the skin is healed.

· *Case histories* ·

Here are some personal accounts of adults with eczema.

· PAUL ·

When I was very young I used to wake up in the morning stuck to the bedclothes in various places. Sometimes the only way to get me moving was to soak the bedsheets off me with warm water. I can remember one morning being taken down to the doctor's surgery on the back of my father's motorbike and I was unable to straighten my arms or my legs during the whole trip. In those days I was in a foetal position for most of the time.

I went to school wearing pyjamas under my clothes. It was the only way round the problem. It kept the blood off my shirt and it was easier to scratch and know that the blood was going on my pyjamas. Now modern man has two buttons open at the top, a hairy chest, medallion and no vest, people ask me why I wear a vest and I say it absorbs the blood. When I say that it cuts them dead and they don't ask any more.

Sometimes I went to school with occlusion bandages on. This is the practice of applying plastic tubular bags over various parts of the body. Ointment is liberally applied on the skin. Then a layer of Tubegauz is put on. Next goes the plastic occlusion, which is sealed at both ends with sticky plaster tape. A final layer of Tubegauz is then applied to finish off the job. When the plastic at the top and the bottom was sealed it blew up like a balloon and it was quite difficult to get clothes on over the top of that. I looked a bit like Michelin Man. It was very hot which was why I scratched it, and then when I scratched a hole in it, boy did it smell, especially if it had been on for three or four days!

When I started getting eczema on my head, discos were really out of the question because when I was a teenager the 'in' light was ultra violet. If you've got seborrhoeic dermatitis of any sort, anything to do with the scalp, the little white flakes glow brilliant mauve a treat. So a head full of scabs is not so good.

When I was bandaged up most weekends I wasn't exactly Mr Universe. Generally I don't think I was of a mind for approaching girls. I didn't feel right. I didn't feel clean. I am certainly much more confident now.

I had a hedge around my garden and my mother was going on at me something silly to cut the hedge because I couldn't go out in the garden – I used to scratch myself after about five minutes. I couldn't cut lawns or do anything. This hedge had been growing for years.

Anyway I went out on a hot summer's day wearing just a pair of shorts, and I cut this hedge. I was getting all dusty and dirty and it was wonderful – nothing was happening. Then I came in at dinner time and I had tomatoes on toast and a cup of tea and I went back out again after an hour or so and after about ten minutes I was scratching myself silly. So I had to retire. I thought about what I had been eating – tomatoes! I had a RAST test and I came out positive to oranges and tomatoes, and also to chicken and eggs. From then on I improved.

A few years ago I joined the naturist movement. I enjoy being naked. To show people 'this is me' and for them not to run away, call me names or treat me as an alien being is such a change. Naturists don't say anything to me about my skin. I am very heavily scarred which shows in the summer where I've got these big white blotches. In the winter I go mauve. But the eczema is now fairly well under control.

I've always had eczema and that makes me different to people who contract it later on. Their motivation for getting better is very different to mine. I'm always comparing myself to what I was yesterday. So are the others, but yesterday they were quite well. I'm building on yesterday, whereas they want to get back to being perfect.

· KERI ·

I've always had bad skin that's taken a long time to heal. I'd been out in the garden kneeling on the grass and just assumed that it was some kind of allergy to that. I didn't have any marks on my skin at all. It was just bright red and on fire is the only way I can describe it. It was horrifyingly itchy. But it hurt to scratch. It burnt me to scratch it. Every joint hurt. I was jumping in and out of the shower. I was in a hot bath at one minute to try and beat the heat and standing under a freezing cold shower the next. It just went on and on and on. Nothing would stop it.

At that stage I didn't know that I had eczema. So I had no creams at all. If I put moisturisers on or baby oil or anything it just burnt like acid. I just couldn't tolerate anything at all. I had a bristle hairbrush which was the hardest thing I could find and I was scratching my legs with that. I would have done anything to stop it. I stood with the shower head on my legs with the water as hot as I could possibly get it. I didn't know what else to do. It was almost as if I burnt it, it would be a different sort of a pain and it wouldn't itch.

I was taking bags of frozen vegetables out of the freezer and I was lying with those on my legs. It was just crazy.

In the end I thought I was going to have a nervous breakdown. It coincided with the weekend and I couldn't get to a doctor. I said to my boyfriend at the time: "What if I've got scabies or something?" I felt so ashamed. By that time I had scratched myself raw and I had blood everywhere. I knew I wasn't dirty but that's how I felt. I felt really contagious. In the end I made an appointment to see my G.P. on the Monday. He said straight away it's eczema and gave me some steroid creams and that was it.

The itching stopped within 24 hours of using the cream. But by that time I was raw and it was really sore then. The skin was very hot but it took the itching away. I could tolerate the heat but I couldn't tolerate the itching. I was on Triludan and Valium for two days as well.

That was when it first started. There have been days when it has just lasted for a 24-hour period. I know when it's going to happen because my skin gets very hot and if I can't get to the steroids within a couple of hours it all starts again.

I am a staff nurse. I must wash my hands about a hundred times a day. Some of the chemicals we use dry my hands and my wrists. It is not worth putting on barrier creams because I'm washing them off again five minutes later. The night before I go to work I put steroids on my hands if there are any dry bits there. Hopefully that sinks in and stops most of the damage and then when I come in from work I give my hands a good scrub and put the creams on again.

I've changed shifts now so I do three long days instead of six short shifts. It doesn't aggravate it so much and if I am in the middle of an inflammation I'll only miss one day at work, or I've only got to work one day and then I've got the next day off. Then it settles down and I can go back. It means I work from 7.30 in the morning to 9 at night three days a week to make up full-time hours.

My arms are scarred a little bit at the elbows but they're not too bad. My legs are quite badly marked and consequently I'm permanently in trousers even if it is 100 degrees outside.

The other side of that is that I broke up with the fellow I was with. When I met somebody else, I didn't have to explain myself, he'd never have known. But we're still together and it came to a time when he saw my legs and that was awful. I felt terrible, but he was brilliant about it.

I have three baths a day if I can manage. I have a minimum of two a day. The main thing I find that helps is emulsifying ointment. I just slap it on with a shovel. Once I've had a bath I just sit there with it on or lie on the bed with a towel and let it all soak in. If I can keep that going twice a day – obviously it depends on the time factor as well – I can hold off an attack for quite a long time.

The worst part is the self-image – what I look like. I understand the condition: I haven't got a problem understanding it or accepting it – but it's what I look like. I'd love to jump into a pair of shorts in the summer but you know that people are looking. The other day at work I had a pair of very fine stockings on and you could see the *marks on my legs. Somebody asked me if I'd been in a car crash. I thought, "I don't need that."*

I think expense is another thing that shocked the hell out of me. When I contacted the National Eczema Society they were talking to me about cotton sheets and duvets and all these kinds of things. I've had to change the bedroom carpet because it was fluffy and I had to buy a new duvet and a new load of bedding and the drugs themselves are quite expensive. My towels were part nylon so I had to change those to 100 percent cotton. I think I paid out nearly £500 in the first couple of weeks. And clothes – there are some clothes I can't wear because they drive me to distraction after an hour or so.

· ANNIE ·
(aged 23, not her real name)

I think it first happened when I was about two years old. It was on the backs of my knees and on my arms. Generally it wasn't that severe but occasionally it would flare up. It went away when I was 11 and came back when I was about 14 years old.

This time it was on my face and that really bothered me. It was very red. I felt awkward and I couldn't really look people in the eye. I was totally obsessed by how it looked. I thought everyone could see it. It restricted my freedom a lot because I felt I couldn't stay over at friends' houses. I was scared it might get worse during the night and then I'd have to face everybody in the morning. I just didn't have any confidence in my appearance. I think if I hadn't had the eczema I would have done a lot more to my appearance instead of trying to hide myself away. I used to try and put my hair over my face and not look up.

When I was taking my A levels it got a lot worse. I think it was the stress. My whole face was covered and it was totally raw and weeping and it went all the way down my neck and on to my chest and my back. It was like that for quite a few months. Once I knew I'd passed my exams and everything was all right there was a slight improvement.

I had started to see a hypnotherapist around the time of my exams. My skin was bright red and weepy at this time. We did relaxation work. We also looked into the psychological causes of the eczema and how it made me feel. It was obviously related to stress. We thought of different ways to work against the habit of scratching and also ways to stop thinking about eczema so much of the time.

During the hypnotherapy one of the first things we did was to look at what the eczema was and I was asked to describe what the eczema looked like. In my head it was like a black cloud hanging over me. The hypnotherapist asked me to find something within myself that cared for my body and wanted it to be healthy and I pictured this flower. Also we made a pact with the eczema. We said to it we will either go down the old path, which is just scratching and giving in to it, or we could try a new path and change.

Another exercise we did was to put the eczema into a box and in our minds we sailed down to the ocean and then put a weight on the box and it sank to the bottom of the sea.

At home when I got itchy I'd try and relax and picture something positive. I made up a garden in my head and did the whole process of getting into the garden. I'd bathe in a cool pool in the imaginary garden to cool my skin down and I'd imagine a cool breeze on my face – that kind of thing. I found it quite hard to do because it was difficult to convince myself that it would work, but you really just try and get lost in a daydream and it can calm you down. If you feel you are going to give in and start scratching again you try and bring these images up instead.

I'd visualise myself scratching and then I would go backwards in my head until I got to the point where I had the idea to scratch and then I'd say to myself, "Stop," and in my mind I'd get up and do something else. It's a difficult thing to do but it actually does work. Sometimes I'd try as many as ten times before I'd actually do it.

After my exams I didn't do much for a few months apart from see the hypnotherapist because I was just so embarrassed about my skin. But I eventually found a job working as a cashier on a till somewhere. When I started I had a big list of things I had to bring with me to work: my creams, of course, and I had a water spray which I filled with spring water. I used to spray this on my face to cool my skin down because it was so hot all the time.

By the time I left work to go to college a few months later my skin was perfect. It was incredible. It was the first time it had been perfect in years. I think working in an unstressed environment where I was totally occupied all day helped a lot. I didn't have time to think about scratching. The hypnotherapy also helped me a good deal.

The first year at university I had emotional problems and I got behind in my work. So the stress of all that brought the eczema back again.

In the summer after the first year I got my old job back again. I worked there for about two months or so and my skin was perfect again. The last two years of college were virtually eczema free.

I graduated last summer and came back home. Nowadays I have a few mild patches of eczema on my face but I don't scratch them at all even though they do itch. It's as if I've trained myself not to.

· SHEILA ·

My hands have always looked very old. When I was in my twenties I went to a skin specialist. He said: "I must have a picture of this lady's hands." He had a nurse about the same age as I was and we had a photo taken together. My husband says my age is now catching up with my hands.

The eczema started when I was 12 years old. It was just after the start of my periods and just after I'd had my ears pierced. It was like elephant's skin. I have been very bad with it. I can remember wanting to hide in a hole. It was at its worst when I was a teenager.

I take evening primrose oil. I also have emulsifying baths which are a nuisance. I don't feel very glamorous. I'm always wrapping up in a big towelling gown. When I come out of the bath I apply steroid cream and petroleum jelly. I can't sit on the settee because of the grease. I have to put a cotton gown on or lay a cotton sheet over the chair.

I can remember when we were first married my husband had to apply Betnovate *cream to me three times a day. I say to my husband: "You just get up, have a shower and put your clothes on. I've love to know what that feeling is like."*

I usually bathe at night. The eczema is not weepy now but it gets red and hot and I use calamine lotion which leaves me looking white and patchy. In the morning I just try and wash the essential bits because my skin gets hot and burning again.

I don't sweat. I feel if I could sweat it would be better.

I haven't done a lot of things I've wanted to do. I don't swim because it stings. My husband is in the scouts and I used to run the Beavers. Beavers don't go camping but the organisers can go to scout camp. I can't go because there are no baths and if there are showers they're very basic. I always feel guilty. I feel other women can go and I can't. I'm told that they can provide a bucket in my tent, but there's no way I can take an emulsifying bath in a bucket!

I get very tired. I get crabby when I'm tired and that sets my skin off. I'm more itchy in the evenings. It's not as flaky and dry as it used to be, now that I'm taking evening primrose oil. I used to have to vacuum the bed when I got up it was so flaky.

I'm not a very good sleeper: I get very, very hot – like I'm going to blow a gasket. My husband says I make him feel seasick, sometimes, with all the scratching which shakes the bed.

I have been using steroid creams for 32 years now. I know that they can harm my body, but it seems to be the only way that I can exist. I am very restricted in the materials that I can wear so I cannot choose many of the fashions or glamorous clothes.

My eczema problems are exacerbated by my frequent severe migraine attacks and asthma. At the moment life is not much fun.

8

THE OVER SIXTIES

An increasing number of people are getting eczema very late in life. Recently a distressed phone call to the National Eczema Society revealed that the caller was experiencing eczema for the first time at the age of 80.

Why there are more people with eczema in the older age group now than ever before is not known. It could be the result of the stresses and strains of modern living. Of course men and women are living longer now and therefore there are many more people in the over-60 age group than there used to be. Also, as the skin grows older, it becomes more vulnerable to the effects of the outside environment, so there are more older people around with thinner and more fragile skin living in a deteriorating environment. Looked at that way it doesn't seem so surprising. What is sad is that there is so little research being done in this growth area.

Stress also has an important part to play. Old age can take an enormous amount of getting used to. Giving up work is not always the pleasure cruise it seems.

One of the reasons that eczema can strike in old age is that was we grow older the skin gets drier. It flakes and can become itchy and sore especially if you scratch. The way to counteract this is to keep the skin moist with regular applications of emollients.

Protect yourself from weather extremes which can be drying to the skin. You probably cover up when you go out in the cold and windy conditions, but are you still a sun lover? Older skin does not fare well with the sun and you really should protect yourself from it. You may also be taking medicines regularly for conditions like arthritis and water retention which make the skin sensitive to strong sunlight and can lead to the development of eczema.

Please read the previous chapter on adult eczema as most of the points mentioned there apply to older people too. Also the chapters on *Keeping Eczema at Bay* (Chapter 9), and *Treatments* (Chapter 12). In the meantime, here are some quick pointers to get you started.

· *Daily routine* ·

Add a little oil to the bath water, but be specially careful as it can make the bath slippery. If you are particularly worried about falling, don't put oil in the bath, just go on to the next stage. Do not use bubble bath instead as this can dry the skin. You should also switch to a soap-substitute (Chapter 12).

The next stage is to apply emollient to the skin which helps reverse the dry skin condition (see Chapter 12). If you have been prescribed a steroid cream, apply this first, to the affected areas only, before you apply the emollient.

Try and remember to apply the emollient at least two or three times a day. Keeping your skin soft and supple is, on a day-to-day basis, the most important part of your management of the condition. This is particularly important if you have eczema on your hands which is often due to dry skin. Keep them well moisturised and wear warm gloves (but not woollen ones) when you go out of doors.

Apart from atopic eczema which is the subject of Chapter 2 and the major part of this book, there are different types of the condition which can occur in later life (see Chapter 11). *Asteatotic eczema* and *varicose eczema* may be of particular interest to you.

· *Personal stories* ·

· ANTHONY ·

As a child I had what my mother used to call 'spots' on my skin which were highly irritant. Whether that was eczema or not I don't know. But I had nothing from then until I retired and I've had it ever since.

It started in a small way on my arms and then it has got gradually worse. At one time my body was covered with eczema – not my face usually. It wasn't weeping. It seemed to be under the skin. But it was highly irritant especially at night. Once or twice I prayed that I might die if I couldn't be cured, it was so dreadful.

I was put on to Prednisolone *tablets with the use of* Dermovate *and* Eumovate *creams. The steroids would damp it down considerably if not entirely at times. But of course they have side effects. They thin the skin and cause swelling of the face. But I was between the devil and the deep blue sea, either having the tablets or having this torment all the time.*

Not being able to sleep at night weakened me considerably and cut down on my activities. The steroid tablets lower one's resistance to infection so I kept getting viral infections. My entire health was lowered. It has completely spoilt my retirement.

But it's been better lately. I've been seeing a dermatologist at Guy's Hospital in London. He's brought me great relief. He's almost got rid of it. He's put me on Zirtex *by day (a non-sedative antihistamine) and* Phenergan *by night. I also have injections of* Synacthen *about every four days. That helps the body to make its own steroids. I've been able to come off the steroid tablets as a result of this.*

I am now able to get on with my life. It has freed me largely of the irritation and I've been very thankful for that.

· PATRICIA ·

My very first experience of eczema was when I was somewhere around the age of 12. It was pretty bad and was on my face and head and on my chest. It was very noticeable.

The eczema didn't disrupt my schooling because it was during the war and school wasn't normal. I lived near Croydon aerodrome and we were in and out of shelters most of the time.

When the eczema was really bad some years later I found the worst thing was other people's reaction to it. They always think it's infectious. If they sit next to you they look at your ghastly hands and at your face and then they immediately move away.

It's affected my life when it's been really bad because I haven't been able to do some of the things I would have done. Since I retired from teaching, I've worked for the Citizens Advice Bureau and when it has been really red and painful I've had to wear gloves just to keep the emollients on my hands, and to prevent myself to some extent from scratching.

There are lots of things I never could do or would do. I never went dancing or swimming. I never did anything which brought me into the close proximity of people. I played tennis but then you were pretty well at the other end of the court.

I think I've missed out a great deal – particularly in meeting the opposite sex. Most people met in the cinema which I couldn't tolerate because of the smoke. Also a lot of people met at dances. The rest of my friends met at the Young Conservatives which wasn't much different, because they went in for dancing and parties, at that time.

I had a very bad attack in my mid-twenties which was caused by lipstick. I used to use a lipstick for sensitive skins but then I couldn't get the colour I wanted. It was for a new red dress – I wanted a matching lipstick. There was only one that matched and I bought it. It was 18 months before we discovered it was the lipstick that set off the eczema as it never affected my lips. But we did find it started to ease off when I stopped using the lipstick. It took between three and six months to clear.

I stayed virtually clear of a really bad attack – just keeping it under control on my hands and face by not using perfumes and very little make-up – all the usual things – until the summer of 1989 when I was extensively affected. It took 18 months to discover it was

*caused by an optical brightener in a wash powder – for those with
sensitive skins. I'm told I'm pretty rare to react to optical
brighteners but I am now sun sensitive.*

9

KEEPING ECZEMA AT BAY

We know that atopic eczema is an inherited condition. Somewhere in their genetic make-up people with eczema have acquired a predisposition to the condition which is often triggered as a result of an allergic reaction. In an ideal world you would test for allergy and avoid the allergen but in real life it is not so easy. However, many of these triggers are known to commonly affect people with eczema. Here are the most common allergens together with tips on how to avoid them.

· *House dust mites* ·

These microscopic creatures are related to spiders and ticks. They are about a third of a millimetre long and so are not visible to the naked eye. They are found, in their millions, in every home, no matter how clean. The house dust mite is the single most important allergy provoker in Britain. They are particularly prolific in damp climates such as ours. They feed on the dead skin flakes that human beings shed constantly. Since people with eczema shed more skin flakes than others, they are a source of constant nourishment to these creatures.

House dust mites thrive on moist and warm environments and live in mattresses, carpets, settees and soft furnishings of all sorts. It is thought that there is a specific protein in house dust mite droppings which is the main cause of the allergy.

House dust mites have a life-span of about six weeks. During this time each female can produce anything up to 80 eggs. It takes between three to four weeks for the eggs to develop into fully fledged adults. So you can see why they are so numerous and so difficult to eradicate. Each adult house dust mite can produce around 30 or 40 faecal droppings per day which is probably what makes them such a major allergy factor for people with eczema. Although you cannot eliminate them entirely from your home, it makes sense to cut down on their presence and protect yourself as much as possible. By the way, they are at their most numerous in autumn, so if you find that your eczema is worse at that time, it could be that house dust mites are a significant provocation for you.

Here are some ways of controlling these creatures:

Bedding

● Mattresses are a major home for house dust mites. If you are buying a new mattress you may like to know that you can buy one with a special interliner in it which protects against house dust mites and their droppings. It is made by Slumberland for their Health Seal Range. Solid foam mattresses are better than interior sprung, Kapok mattresses are the worst and water beds are the least likely to be colonised by house dust mites.

Cover existing mattresses with airtight plastic covers which are available by mail order. Alternatively you can enclose the mattress in a liner. Both these methods act as a barrier between you and house dust mites and are an effective way of keeping the dust mite and its droppings at bay. These covers are easy to keep clean. Mail order houses which supply both are advertised widely. The Intervent interliners as well as the Slumberland Health Seal range are available in some of the larger Boots stores.

● Bedding should be of man-made and washable fibres rather than natural fibres: this includes duvets and pillows. Wash sheets and pillowcases daily and duvets about once a week. Wash in temperatures as hot as the fabric washing instructions will allow. Anti-allergy pillows and duvets which you can wash in very hot temperatures are available, as are plastic covers or interliners to cover duvets and pillowcases. But be careful using plastic covers with young children as there is a risk of suffocation. Slumberland also sell pillows with interliners incorporated into them. If you use these you will not need to wash the bedding so frequently, but you will need to wipe over plastic covers with a damp cloth.

Regularly air pillows, duvets and mattresses and expose them to sunlight to kill house dust mites. Remove all feather bedding and pillows.

● Soft toys are a major living ground for the house dust mite. If your child has eczema try and cut down on the amount of these toys that he or she has if you cannot eliminate them altogether, and try and discourage them from being kept on the bed. If this is not possible, wash the toys every week. In addition put the toys into plastic bags and place in the freezer for five or six hours (or more) and then give them a machine wash.

● Padded headboards should be avoided as they are difficult to keep dust-free.

Bedrooms

Carpets are great gatherers of dust, particularly bedroom carpets where the humidity is likely to be higher. So wooden floors, lino or tiles are probably better particularly if they are vacuumed or damp-dusted daily. Dispense with rugs or if you must have them, make sure they are small, light and easily washable.

To keep furnishing simple and easy to clean have as few ornaments as you possibly can without feeling bereft. Have plain wood or plastic chairs instead of upholstered ones.

Textured wallpaper, wall hangings and plants can also collect dust and fungi. Dried flowers, especially, are great dust gatherers and so are books.

Store luggage and outdoor clothing out of the bedroom and make sure that clothing and toys are put away in a cupboard and the door is kept shut.

Choose curtains or blinds that are easy to wash, rather than heavy fabrics. Venetian blinds collect a lot of dust so avoid these, fabric blinds that you can damp-dust are better.

Treat all beds in the same room identically. Bunk beds for children with eczema should be avoided but if there is no choice, the top bunk is preferable for an eczematous child as the dust mite droppings in the mattress above can come through to the sleeper below.

Cleaning

Always damp-dust as dry-dusting releases the mite droppings into the atmosphere. All surfaces should be damp-dusted at least once a week. If you have eczema, wear PVC gloves with cotton inner gloves for any washing and cleaning.

Vacuuming is preferable to sweeping. Do this regularly, preferably with a cleaner especially designed for people with dust allergy. If your mattress does not have a plastic cover, you will need to vacuum that too.

Most conventional vacuum cleaners will retain virtually all the large dust particles but the sub-microscopic particles leak through the filter system and become airborne and settle on the furniture. These airborne particles of house dust mite droppings trigger allergies in the shape of eczema, asthma, rhinitis and so on. The vacuum cleaner also becomes clogged with the dust it collects so each time you switch on the cleaner, dust particles are released into the room. You may find it helpful to wear a mask. Also make sure that the cleaner has a strong suction and that the bags do not leak. Change the bags frequently and keep any members of the family who have eczema out of the room while you are vacuuming.

There is a medical vacuum cleaner which boasts an absolute dust filtration system and conforms to British Standards 5415 Section 2.2. It has filtration in accordance with the Supplement No.1. Called

Medivac, a filtration certificate is supplied with each machine which apparently proves a very high rate of filtration. Electrolux also produces a vacuum cleaner with an advanced air filtration system. *Electrolux Airstream 1000* is an upright vacuum cleaner with a greater suction power than other uprights. It has a special dust bag to prevent the discharge of dust back into the air.

Carpet shampooing machines are not thought to be of any help in reducing the house dust mite population. Most leave a small residue of water behind in the carpet pile and this added humidity may in fact encourage these creatures to increase and multiply!

Other rooms

In other rooms you do not have to be quite so stringent as you are not likely to be spending as much time in them as bedrooms.

Again, carpeting is not the best option, but if that is what you like, choose man-made fibres rather than wool. People with eczema should avoid sitting for any length of time directly on a carpeted floor, but when they do they should sit on a small cotton sheet or towel.

A wooden chair in the bedroom can look rather fetching, but in a lounge you may want something a bit more luxurious. Aim always for furnishing that is easy to wash or to clean regularly. Work out a compromise between what appeals to you aesthetically and what you can cope with cleaning daily. Curtains, again, will need regular cleaning, so choose ones that are not going to be too troublesome or expensive.

Heating

Remember that temperature control in people with eczema does not function as well as in people without the condition. So do not over-heat rooms as this can trigger the eczema. Equally, don't let the house get too cold and damp as the eczematous person will not be wearing close-fitting woollies.

Minimise damp

Avoid humidifiers and vaporisers, repair leaky pipes, defective walls and roofs and make sure there is a damp proof course if possible. Extractor fans in kitchens and bathrooms are also a good investment because they tend to reduce the condensation which encourages both house dust mites and moulds. Keeping the air as dry as possible is the best way of keeping dust mites at bay but, having said that, ducted air heating is not a good idea because when you switch it on it can blow dust particles around the room. Anti-allergy dehumidifiers can also be helpful.

If you are buying a house, try and make sure that it is not damp. Avoid buying one that is near open water or an undergrown stream. Remember that older houses are usually more difficult to dust than newer ones.

· *Pets* ·

Although they are a very desirable part of family life, dogs, cats, horses, rabbits, birds and other animals are very likely to trigger eczema. Almost any furry pet can produce an allergic reaction in someone with the condition. It is worth knowing that the allergy may not show itself straight away. It often takes time before you start reacting to the animal and the build-up can become so intense that you cannot enter a room which has housed a cat or a dog without reacting to it. Pets that are kept in the home shed their dander all over the house so virtually every room is affected. Please see Chapter 4 for more information on pets.

· *Tobacco smoke* ·

According to the National Eczema Society, banning cigarette smoking from your house is probably the most significant measure you can take. Many of the substances released in tobacco smoke can irritate the eyes, nose and lungs. Furthermore, exposure to this smoke increases the chances of new allergies developing.

· *Pollen* ·

Grass pollens, together with some tree pollens, are particularly troublesome to people with eczema. But since pollination is a seasonal event, you can get some idea as to whether or not you are affected. If you find that your eczema is particularly bad between the beginning of April and the end of May it is likely to be tree pollen that is affecting you since trees pollinate at this time.

However, if the bad times come a little later on – between the beginning of May and the end of July, you are probably allergic to grass pollen. You can, of course, be susceptible to both.

Keeping your windows shut at home, at work and in the car during the day is a must. Don't sit on grass or do any gardening during this time. Don't even think about mowing the lawn. If someone else is doing it, make sure all windows and doors are kept shut and remain so for some hours afterwards.

If you do come into contact with pollen, shower off immediately and wash your hair as well. Afterwards, rub yourself liberally with emollients and keep doing so until your skin feels soft and supple again.

· *Fungi and moulds* ·

The spores from moulds and fungi can cause allergic reactions in people with eczema. These exist in rooms with rising damp but also can be found in dark, humid and poorly ventilated areas where there is heavy condensation. They also live on food like beans and grains, dried fruit and apples. Mould also appears on plants, trees and compost heaps.

Avoid storing large quantities of mould-gathering foods. If you do have mould-laden objects, keep them well dusted.

Keeping the house well-ventilated is also important. Funnily enough this is more of a problem in modern houses which are well insulated than in older housing which usually allows constant circulation of air. Not only can poor ventilation encourage the growth of moulds and fungi, it can give rise to a contaminated household atmosphere which, in turn, can irritate the skin, eyes, nose and lungs. Poor ventilation can also increase humidity which we now know is just what house dust mites like!

But of course life isn't that simple and leaving windows wide open when the pollen count is high, or there is pollution in the air, is not a good idea. A useful compromise during the high pollen season may be to keep the windows open at night and closed during the day.

Air filters can be very effective in reducing the build-up of pollen and mould spores, particularly in bedrooms. However, only the 'high efficiency' particle air filter systems are recommended because ordinary filtering systems do not remove particles quickly enough when clouds are released during vacuuming, bed making and other such household chores.

· *Laundry products* ·

Trial and error is usually the best way to discover which washing powder and liquids you can tolerate and which you cannot. But there are some general guidelines:

● Biological powders and liquids which contain enzymes are thought to cause itchiness and irritation in people with eczema. It is usually best to go for the non-biological variety.

● Fabric conditioners that contain perfume can also cause problems if you are sensitive to perfumes. There are some that are non-perfumed or contain very little perfume which you may be able to tolerate.

● Laundry products that contain bleach can cause irritation. Many heavy-duty laundry powders contain bleaches but the liquids do not.

● Green products may be environmentally friendly but may not be so good for you. If they contain enzymes or perfume, you would probably do best to give them a miss.

● Once you have settled on a product that suits you, all should be plain sailing until you spot the words 'new' or 'improved'. In this case examine the contents carefully to make sure that the newness doesn't include the ingredients you want to avoid.

● Make sure that you do not use more powder or liquid in the wash than is needed. Amounts will vary according to whether or not you live in a hard or soft water area, so follow recommendations given on the packets.

● If you are sensitive to laundry powders or liquids, it is a good idea to give your washing an extra rinse.

● When hand washing it is very important to ensure that all the detergent is removed from the garment. Keep rinsing until the water runs clear. If you have eczema protect your hands by wearing rubber or PVC gloves with a pair of cotton inners.

· *Clothing* ·

Tight-fitting, heavy clothing or material that doesn't allow the skin to breathe can make you hot and itchy. Nylon, polyesters and woollens can also promote the itch. Cotton is the safest choice of clothing material for anyone with eczema, apart from cotton that has been treated to be crease-resistant.

Although, as a rule of thumb, 100 percent cotton is the best buy, there are fabric mixes that many people with eczema can wear quite happily. So try cotton and polyester, viyella, silk or a soft acrylic.

Feel is quite a good yardstick to go by. If a fabric feels soft to the touch it will probably be all right for you. Watch out for possible irritants in the shape of rough seams, elastic, labels, and metal clips and zip fastenings which may rub. If they are made of nickel, you may be allergic to them.

Make sure that you wear cool, loose-fitting, preferably 100 percent cotton clothing when the weather is hot. In winter, wear cotton clothes next to your skin and put wool, or other warm fabrics on top.

Dyes and finishes can cause *allergic contact eczema*. A good practice is to wash new clothes before wearing them because this gets rid of the finish or the excess dye. However, some people are allergic to strong colour dyes and may have to avoid wearing them next to the skin.

The National Eczema Society has a fairly comprehensive list of cotton goods stockists and suppliers of house dust mite prevention bedding, so you may like to get in touch with them.

· *Diet* ·

Food allergy does not seem to be a major cause of eczema with adults, allergy to artificial colourings and preservatives is more common. But some people do find that certain foods such as nuts and fish can trigger the condition. Stimulants like coffee, tea, alcohol, chocolate, tobacco as well as some drugs can make you itchy. Some adults do find that dairy food is a problem in which case switching to goat's milk, or sheep's milk or soya milk is a good idea, but it is very seldom that the condition can be brought under control through diet alone.

The best way to test for food allergy is by trial and error. Keep a diary of what you eat and note any reactions. You may need to do this over several months to get a definite pattern. Some people try and do it in retrospect, by thinking back to what they ate as soon as they get very itchy or experience a flare-up of the condition. There are reasons why this does not work very well. Firstly, it may not be what you ate that set off the itching but may, instead, be one of the environmental factors we have already discussed. Secondly, you don't always get a reaction to what you have eaten straight away. Thirdly, memory is far from infallible and you may remember every constituent of your four-course meal but forget the couple of gulps you had of someone else's orange drink, or the sweet you popped into your mouth on your way out of the house.

Don't go on elimination diets or cut out important foods without medical collaboration, either with your doctor or a qualified dietitian. The importance of dairy food is very obvious for children but remember calcium is necessary for adolescents and adults too.

Keep to as varied a diet as possible. If you have a very restricted diet you could find yourself becoming allergic to the foods you eat. Fresh food, particularly fresh fruit and vegetables, is very important in keeping you healthy and your skin itch-free. (See Chapter 4.)

10

TRAVEL AND HOLIDAYS

One of the main problems about a condition like eczema is that it can have such a restricting effect on your life. The excitement of going abroad or even visiting pastures new in your own country can be very much dampened if you're worried about heat, dust, clothing, bedding and diet – to name but a few considerations.

But holidays and travel can have advantages particularly to a person with eczema. You can use this time to test limits which you may not be able to do at home.

Many people find that when they go abroad and meet the sun or experience days of relaxation that their eczema does improve or even magically disappears.

As ever, the rule with eczema is to be well aware that you have it and may need to treat it. Choosing the location is often the starting point of holiday plans and it is important to keep your skin in mind here. Most people with atopic eczema find that their condition improves in the sun.

People with *photosensitive eczema* however should steer clear of the sun. Also some antihistamines can make your skin very sensitive to sunlight. If you regularly take antihistamines, before you plan your holiday ask your doctor if the one you take causes photosensitivity.

In any event, getting hot can make you very itchy and that in turn can aggravate the eczema. So a good location would be somewhere sunny but not too hot. If you are sensitive to pollens you are likely to be happier in a seaside location rather than a country one and if animals affect your skin stay away from farm holidays. If you do want a countryside holiday, take extra emollients, steroid creams and antihistamines just in case the eczema gets worse.

Are you on a restricted diet? If so, you might find self-catering holidays the simplest to organise, or look out for hotels and guest houses that cater for special diets. Self-catering is also good for anyone worried about bedding. You can take your own anti-dust-mite bedding with you and you can change the sheets as often as you would at home (if there is a washing machine available.) Another advantage to self-catering is that you don't have to worry about getting creams or blood on the sheets if they are your own.

Many people, whether they have eczema or not, behave in a very different way when they are on holiday. It's easier to 'let your hair down' so to speak, and it's easier to try things out or test limits with people you are unlikely to ever see again in a place you need never come back to.

If you are normally too shy to speak to people because they may reject you, a holiday is a good time to try a little bit of assertiveness. If the people you talk to are nice, it's a positive experience that will stimulate your self-confidence and enhance your holiday: if they're not, to heck with them – who were they anyway?

Equally, it can be a good time to test for skin reactions. Maybe you don't swim at home because you found that the water stung or your eczema flared up. On holiday you can try again. Use plenty of emollient beforehand to act as a barrier and slap it on again afterwards. It may be that you are not so sensitive now; or it may be that if you keep trying you will find a means of coping. If you find the water still affects you, at least you don't have to go to work the next day or attend some social function so you can cope with the flare-up in a laid-back way.

· *Your skin in the sun* ·

Whether or not a person has eczema over-exposure to the sun can have harmful effects. The sun also has a very drying effect on the skin and you will need to use much more in the way of emollients in sunny climates than you do otherwise.

The colour and type of your skin dictates how much sunbathing you can do but you must always introduce your skin to the sun a little at a time and build up resistance and tan gradually. The rest of the time you should keep your skin covered by wearing loose cotton clothing and a wide-brimmed sun hat.

If you have a very pale skin which burns easily and never tans it is best to stay out of the sun, but people with this skin type are rare. More usual is the pale skin which tans with difficulty (and then only slightly) but burns easily. You must be careful with this type of skin. Always use a sunscreen with a high Sun Protection Factor of 15 or more. Never go out into the sun without it and apply it every two hours or so. Always re-apply the sunscreen after you have been swimming even if it is water-resistant. People with darker skins can usually get away with a SPF 10 sunscreen but it is much better to stick with a higher SPF than take chances with a lower one.

Cracked skin can sting like mad in the sea but rather than give swimming a miss altogether, try and apply a liberal amount of emollient beforehand as a barrier and enter the sea gradually. You might find the stinging settles down and the salt may even have a healing effect. Afterwards make sure that you wash very carefully to remove any residual salt and sand. And don't forget to put on plenty of emollient.

If you can find a holiday location with a pool that uses a more eczema-friendly disinfectant than chlorine, that is ideal, but even with chlorine, it is worth trying the barrier method with emollient to see if it will work for you. Don't stay too long in the pool to start off with, and don't forget to shower or bathe afterwards and re-apply the creams.

If the skin is a little sore or itchy, use a mild steroid cream. If it is at all pink from the sun, the steroid cream will help, but keep your skin covered for the next couple of days. Don't use after-sun lotions as many of these contain antihistamines which can cause allergic reactions (see Chapter 12).

Here are some reminders:

Tips for travel and holidays

● Take extra emollients, steroid creams and antihistamines. Pack them in a hard plastic container to stop them from oozing out.
● Don't forget the sunscreens.
● Remember to take extra cotton clothing.
● If you are self-catering, take extra bedding. Don't forget your washing-up and cleaning gloves.
● Don't forget to take your special washing powders and soap-substitutes.
● If you are on a diet, make lists of what you need to take and then take extra.
● It is always useful to take a list of your medications with you together with your NHS number. If you are travelling in Europe take the appropriate medical forms (E111).
● In a hot climate keep creams in the fridge so they feel nice and cool when applied.
● For hot, itchy skin, fill a plastic bag with ice cubes and place next to the skin for instant relief.
● Use plenty of barrier creams (vaseline is a good one) before you go swimming.
● A tepid shower or bath after swimming is a must and re-apply a liberal amount of emollient.
● Sun hats, sun umbrellas and a sun canopy over a pram or push-chair are important items to take with you.
● A cotton sheet spread over the car seat can stop you from feeling hot and sticky, but make sure that the seat belt remains effective.

· *NES holidays* ·

The National Eczema Society, in conjunction with the National Asthma Campaign, runs a series of holidays during the summer for different age groups. The idea is to bring together young people who have eczema and asthma in a safe, happy environment where they can build up their confidence and social skills through sharing a variety of activities.

Many of these activities are adventurous in anybody's language: canoeing, sailing, windsurfing, orienteering, fencing, archery, cycling, ice skating and dry-skiing to name but a few! Everyone is encouraged to take part in and enjoy these activities knowing that there is medical and nursing support constantly available. The aim is to help the holiday makers put the eczema or asthma to one side and get on with enjoying themselves in this vigorous and exciting sort of way. Not only does it encourage people who may have lived under the shadow of their condition to come out of their shells in this controlled and caring atmosphere, but it also helps teach them that they can do these kind of things because if there are consequences they can cope with them. It can have a very liberating effect.

There was one young lad of 15 who recently went on an NES holiday. He was very nervous. He had never been away from home before. He had never been on holiday because he felt different and was worried about all the creams he had to put on. He had been bullied consistently at school because of his skin and his self-image was very poor.

Prior to the holiday he rang a few times saying he couldn't swim and he didn't want to do this and that. He didn't want to share a room with anyone because he itched during the night and he had to get up and scratch and it disturbed everybody. He didn't want anyone to look at his skin. The holiday organiser wrote and explained that everyone shared rooms. He was grouped with another boy of about the same age who had eczema and the two got on very well. The boy blossomed. He arrived very introverted and yet became one of the leaders on the holiday. He found that no one bothered or minded. He could relax and be himself – very sociable and out-going – given half a chance!

Each holiday lasts a week and is closely supervised by a holiday leader who heads a team of helpers, many of whom have first-hand experience of either eczema and/or asthma. In addition there are nurses and a doctor. Each holiday group comprises about 30 holidaymakers and about 14 or 15 helpers who are on hand 24 hours a day to provide encouragement, support and advice. Emphasis is placed on health education and the medical staff run sessions on eczema and asthma and their practical management, including relaxation and breathing techniques, inhaler and medication use and the application of emollients and steroid creams.

With such a large ratio of helpers to holiday makers, even the youngest can be encouraged to try new activities. One little boy of eight always slept with bandages on. He was adamant that he wasn't going to go near the swimming pool even though it was a nice pool area with a slope so that people could enter the pool gradually. All the young ones went in, and eventually he had a go. The helpers put lots of *Diprobase* cream on him before he went in and he was fine.

Another child had very bad eczema on his back. It was noticeably worse if he got stressed or if he got very hot. So the helpers would take a couple of spare T-shirts for him when they went on an outing, together with some tubes of cream. If he got hot and itchy he would sit down while somebody put cream on his back. He would change his T-shirt which cooled him down and after a little while, when he felt more calm, he would be able to carry on with the activities.

In this way youngsters learn that they don't have to hide from life just because they have eczema. Their condition means that they may have to work a bit harder in looking after themselves but, at the end of the day, they can do the same things as everybody else.

The holidays are divided into three age groups – youngsters from about seven to 12, teenagers, and then young adults up to the age of 30. A wide range of diets are anticipated and catered for.

On-site facilities usually include a swimming pool, games room and craft rooms as well as meeting rooms and playing fields.

Although the emphasis is on fun and encouraging holidaymakers to try new activities, attention is given to providing an atmosphere where people can get to know each other and talk about their condition without the fear of being misunderstood or stigmatised. Many youngsters find it easier to make friendship with members of the opposite sex in an environment where no one is going to turn their noses up at eczematous hands or feel they are going to catch an infection if they come too close.

Young adult holidays are planned on much the same lines where they can take part in the sports activities as and when they want to. However, many find it relaxing to be in the company of other people who have eczema or asthma and to be able to talk about their treatments and problems in a way that they may not be able to do elsewhere.

The holidays are subsidised and some are grant-aided. If you would like to know about them contact the National Eczema Society or the National Asthma Campaign. Addresses of both organisations appear in Chapter 17.

11

INFECTED AND OTHER TYPES OF ECZEMA

· *Infected eczema* ·

Eczema herpeticum

This is a complication of eczema and not a type of eczema but it can be a very serious condition. It is a result of the eczema being infected by the *herpes simplex virus* which is the virus that produces cold sores.

Herpes simplex is one of the most common viruses and is very infectious. Normally cold sores appear around the mouth. They can be very small and often go undetected as they seldom cause undue problems in anyone who does not have eczema. However, in a person with eczema this virus can appear on areas of the skin where the condition exists. It can then enter the bloodstream and spread very quickly to other areas of the eczematous skin as well as the internal organs. This is when it becomes serious and, if not dealt with quickly, it can even be fatal.

Eczema herpeticum appears in little clusters on the skin which look like small blisters. These blisters start off filled with a clear fluid but later turn to pus. The blisters get scratched, become very raw and weepy and start to have a crusted look.

After the first attack of the virus an immunity is usually achieved making it unlikely to be caught again from someone else. But it lingers on in the body and can be re-activated if the person is unwell or sometimes if the skin is exposed to bright sunlight or cold winds.

Children are particularly susceptible to this virus as they may not have built up an immunity, but it can affect all age groups. It is therefore important to recognise it and act quickly.

If the eczema has suddenly got much worse for no reason or if it has changed in look, particularly if you see the small blisters described, seek medical advice immediately. Eczema herpeticum is usually accompanied by a high temperature and the person is singularly lethargic and unwell. One of the problems is that doctors do not always recognise this illness and it is not always diagnosed, so mention the possibility of eczema herpeticum to the doctor.

The patient is often treated in hospital but this is not always necessary. Treatment will usually involve the anti-viral drug *acyclovir.* This can be given by injection, by mouth or in the form of an ointment. (See Joanna's story, Chapter 4.)

It is important that someone with atopic eczema should stay away from skin contact with anyone who has cold sores.

Infected eczema

It is quite common for eczema to become infected with bacteria. Bacteria thrive in moist situations in the outer body and usually these are places like the inside of the nose and the genital area. In someone with eczema there are many more areas in the body for the bacteria to live comfortably since cracked, scratched and broken skin provide just the kind of moist and nutritious environment that they need to thrive. This means that a person with eczema is likely to be housing much more bacteria than his non-eczematous counterpart.

A small amount of bacteria on the body is quite healthy: a large amount is not. When a person is housing bacteria in large quantities they are said to be infected. Added to this is the fact that with non-eczematous people the skin acts as barrier between the internal body and the outside world. When the skin is broken the door is not quite so firmly shut.

The most common bacterial infection is known as *Staphylococcus aureus*. It can cause *impetigo* in people who don't have eczema and can also give rise to boils.

In people with eczema *Staphylococcus aureus* is a frequent cause of a sudden worsening of the eczema. If the eczema has started to spread and is weepy with yellow crusts or pus-filled spots, it could well be that this bacterial infection has started to get out of control. The person may also have a slight temperature and swollen glands and there may be an enlargement of the lymph nodes. The latter are lumps that appear in the groins, armpits or neck area and they exist to filter out bacteria and stop them from entering the bloodstream. Swollen lymph nodes can be painful and tender to the touch. Most people with eczema do have some swollen glands – in the armpits, groins and in the neck. It's nothing to worry about: it's just part of the condition.

When eczema becomes infected in this way it must be treated by a doctor. Oral antibiotics are the most effective and most usual treatment. Sometimes antibiotic ointments are prescribed to treat minor outbreaks of infected eczema.

When oral antibiotics are prescribed it is most important to complete the dose as if you don't, not only can the infection re-occur, but it can also become resistant to the antibiotic, making it much more difficult to treat.

However, better than treatment is prevention. You can help prevent the eczema from becoming infected by keeping the skin clean and supple. Regular moisturising will help keep the skin well sealed and uninviting to bacterial infections.

Remember always to keep containers and tubes of creams and ointments well sealed to avoid introducing bacteria.

Another form of bacterial infection is known as *Group A streptococcus*. This usually appears in the shape of sore throats but occasionally can affect eczematous skin. Again, it needs treating on the off-chance that it leads to a more serious condition like, for example, rheumatic fever. Follow the usual rule of thumb in that if the eczema suddenly gets worse for no known reason, a visit to the doctor is important.

· *Other types of eczema* ·

Irritant contact eczema

This type of eczema is due to physical damage to the skin and can be caused by chemicals or friction or anything which can irritate the skin. The most likely places for it are the hands and feet but it can also appear on the lower arms. It is caused by contact with substances that irritate or damage the skin. People whose work brings them constantly in physical contact with irritants are the most vulnerable and these include hairdressers, nurses and housewives. Agricultural workers, car workers, interior decorators, building workers as well as those dealing in rubber, textile and chemicals can also be vulnerable to irritant contact eczema. There is usually a history of atopic eczema. The kind of substances that can cause this eczema are: *Soap or other detergents, Chemicals, Water, Acids, Alkalis, Solvents, Oils, Soil, Fertilisers, Cement.*

If you can identify the substance that is causing the problem and avoid coming into contact with it, the eczema will be cured, but often this is not possible. The next best thing is to keep the contact to a minimum. You can do this by protecting your hands by wearing rubber gloves with cotton inners when using these substances (but don't keep the gloves on for more than 20 minutes at a time). Use barrier creams and steroid creams when necessary to keep the eczema under control. If it is itchy an antihistamine in tablet or syrup form may help. More information appears under *Hand eczema* in this chapter.

Allergic contact eczema

This is also caused by coming into contact with substances that irritate or damage the skin but here it is an allergic reaction. The sensitivity can build up quite quickly and the rash can spread to another part of the body.

Patch testing is a good way to try and identify the cause. Here are some likely ones:

Nickel (very common in jewellery, particularly earrings and rings. Also appears as fasteners in clothing, studs, zips, suspenders and buckles. Coins and stainless steel also contain nickel). *Rubber* (this can be in gloves, footwear and straps), *Leather, Paints, Cement, Cosmetics, Topical medicine, Antihistamines, Anaesthetics, Lanolin, Plants, Fruit and vegetable skins, Hair dyes, Glues.*

Again defining and avoiding the offending substance is the best treatment as well as the guide lines given in irritant contact eczema. Also read the information given in hand and foot eczema below.

Asteatotic eczema

This can also be referred to as *eczema craquele* and often develops for the first time on the shins. It appears as a result of the thinning and drying of the skin which is why it appears so often in the older age group. So the moisturising routine is especially important in counteracting this condition. Use as soap-substitute and avoid using harsh disinfectants or detergents without wearing protective gloves. The key to handling this condition is to keep the skin as moist and supple as possible.

Discoid eczema

This develops as scaly, itchy, coin-shaped, patches on the limbs which may blister and weep when severe. Again, it is thought to be connected with the drying out of the skin but is also usually associated with bacterial infection. It can be misdiagnosed as ringworm. It occurs more often during winter, with low humidity and central heating. Too much soap can make the condition worse so soap substitutes and regular moisturising are a must. You may also be prescribed a steroid cream or a combination antibiotic and steroid cream to aid healing.

Ear eczema

Different types of eczema affect the ear and there are various causes. Contact eczema, described above, is one. This can be caused by ear-piercing. The nickel in earrings is a well-known cause, so if you are thinking of having your ears pierced make sure the earrings are 9 or 18 carat gold, British sterling silver, or platinum. You can also use hypoallergenic earrings made of plastic or stainless steel and there are nickel-free ear-piercing studs called 'Poly Dots' available (for address see Chapter 17).

Another cause of contact eczema in this area is wearing tight-fitting spectacles, particularly if the frames are made of metal. It can also be caused by shampoos, hair sprays and dyes, perm lotions or medications used in that area of the body. Hearing aids are another possible cause.

Both atopic eczema and seborrhoeic eczema (described below) can affect the ear.

If the eczema is on the outside of the ear you can treat it as normal with creams and ointments. However, eczema inside the ear canal must be treated with caution and you must seek medical advice. If you use cotton buds you need to be extremely careful not to insert them too deep into the ear canal as this can damage the eardrum, and they must be sterile or you may introduce an infection. Never use hard or non-sterile objects to scratch the itch as you can do a great deal of harm. Be particularly careful if you are treating a baby or child.

Scale and ear-wax can be removed by washing out the ear but this must be done under medical supervision. In many G.P. practices the practice nurse is available to provide this service.

Sometimes eczema in the ear can be accompanied by a partial loss of hearing. This is often caused by a build-up of wax or scales in the ear. If you experience this you need to see your doctor.

Foot eczema

This can be caused by *contact eczema* or *pompholyx eczema,* both of which are described in this chapter.

There is also a possibility that you may be allergic to the chromate used to tan the leather with which the shoes are made. Leather is tanned to prevent it from rotting. A large proportion of people who have an allergic reaction to footwear are found to be allergic to chromate. It may be the shoe's adhesive causing the problem. The first step is to get referred to a dermatologist who could arrange a patch test to try and identify the allergy. With this information you could contact SATRA (Shoe and Allied Trades Research Association) who can give you some pointers on the type of footwear to avoid.

The clothing and footwear section of The Disabled Living Foundation may be able to give you up-to-date information that can help you in your search for more suitable footwear.

Here are some general tips:

● Wear socks, stockings or tights that are 100 percent cotton or make sure that they contain a high proportion of cotton.
● Footwear also should allow the foot to breathe, such as leather shoes with leather linings or absorbent in-soles. Plastic footwear, trainers or other shoes that make the feet sweat should be avoided.
● Try not to wear the same shoes every day as this can lead to a build-up of moisture in the leather.
● You may like to try bandaging the feet at night once you have applied the creams or ointments. This will ensure that the medication is well absorbed.

Hand eczema

Contact eczema on the hands is very prevalent and very distressing. Here are some suggestions to keep this condition under control.

● Use a soap-substitute, particularly if you are constantly washing your hands. Dry them gently and thoroughly and always moisturise them afterwards.
● Keep handwashing clothes or other items down to a minimum and whenever possible use plastic or rubber gloves with cotton inners. The same applies to washing your hair.
● If you wear rings remember that any nickel in them could be a problem for you. The safest rings are those made with 18 carat gold, platinum and British Sterling silver. Never wash your hands when wearing a ring and don't keep rings on when you are doing housework.
● Always wear gloves when using polishes, solvents and stain removers.
● Your skin may react to some fruit and vegetables. Wear gloves when handling citrus fruits, garlic, onions, radishes and tomatoes. Cheese can also cause a reaction.
● If you can, wash up in running water and always wear plastic or rubber gloves with cotton inners. If any water enters the glove take it off immediately. Remember not to wear the gloves for too long and wash them regularly in hot water.

Light sensitive eczema

Eczema that is caused by sunlight is rare. When it does occur, the most common sites are the face, backs of the hands and forearms. They become very red, sore and weepy. It can usually be treated quite effectively by using sunscreens with a high SPF factor, but you must first seek medical advice.

This type of eczema can also occur when people are taking medication that interacts with the sunlight. Some antihistamines can do this, as can drugs taken for arthritis and other conditions.

Anti-bacterial substances in special soaps as well as perfumes and cosmetics can also have this effect.

Pompholyx eczema

This can be either on the hands or feet and starts with the development of tiny, itchy blisters. These break and weep and the skin can become inflamed and scaly. It is not known what causes this condition but stress can be a factor. Soaking hands or feet in a solution of potassium permanganate can sometimes be helpful. Also follow the guidelines given for hand and foot eczema.

Seborrhoeic eczema

In adults this type of eczema can be a chronic condition but is usually mild. It is an itchy, scaly condition which appears on the scalp, face, ears, eyelids, eyebrows as well as the upper parts of the body. It can also appear in the groin and tummy button. The eczema can have a red, inflamed look and become crusty.

You need to wear loose fitting cotton clothing as sweating, particularly in the folds of the skin, can aggravate the condition and lead to secondary infection.

Where the scalp is involved, shampoos containing coal tar and salicylic acid are used in place of an ordinary one. If creams are being applied to the scalp it is important to part the hair and rub them well into the scalp to achieve maximum absorption. They can be shampooed off the next day. (For a list of shampoos see Chapter 12.)

You will need to be very careful about the cosmetics you use as the skin will be particularly sensitive to irritants.

Urticaria

This condition is more commonly knows as *hives*, *welts* or *nettle rash*. It is a whitish rash which is very itchy and appears in weals of varying sizes. It often appears in clusters with an outer redness and stinging and burning sensations can accompany the itch. It can last a few hours, weeks or several months and come and go quite suddenly, appearing in different sites on the body at different times.

There are many possible causes for this condition. Stress is one that is not uncommon, particularly in people with a history of atopy. Medicine is another; penicillin, aspirin and codeine being the most common causes. Certain foods can also cause urticaria and these include fish, particularly shellfish, berries, particularly strawberries, eggs, milk, nuts, cheese, yeasts, tomatoes, peppers, spices as well as food additives, particularly azo dyes and benzoates. House dust, pollens, tobacco smoke, mould spores and animal dander can also trigger the condition and if you wear anything tight over a period of time, like elastic, straps, belts and so on, urticaria can result.

Whatever the cause, the substance that is released into the body is *histamine* and it is this that sets off the urticaria. So the obvious treatment is to block off the histamine production and this is done by means of oral antihistamines. However, antihistamine creams should never be used to treat this condition as the skin can become sensitive to them making treatment much more difficult. There is a variety of oral antihistamines available and which one you use is a matter of personal choice. Calamine lotion can help soothe the skin if it is very itchy.

If the condition is caused by stress, try and find a way in which you can unwind and let it go even if it is just for a while. Many people find that taking up a sport is a good one. Vigorous exercise is a good way of getting rid of a build-up of adrenalin in the system. Listening to music or getting involved in a hobby are also good ways of relaxing.

Varicose eczema

This is also known as *stasis* or *gravitational eczema*. The condition appears on the site of varicose veins, particularly on the inside of the ankle. Women are more prone to varicose veins than men and people who are overweight are more likely to get them. If the rash is itchy and burning it may mean that the skin is thinning and this could eventually lead to the development of a leg ulcer.

Support stockings can be very helpful in preventing swelling of the ankles and may also stop the eczema or an ulcer occurring. Standing on your feet all day is not helpful to this condition. Rest with your legs raised as much as you can.

You could also put a soft pad or bandage over the eczema and the varicose vein. This not only gives protection to that sensitive area, but if you add tar or ichthammol paste to the pad or bandage, it will soothe the skin and cut down on the itchiness. It is important to get the condition medically diagnosed and treated.

Vesicular eczema

This is a blistering type of eczema usually affecting the sides of the fingers, palms of the hands and soles of the feet. Later the skin may peel and split. Secondary bacterial infection is common. Nickel sensitivity is thought to be a common cause. Potassium permanganate soaks can ease irritation in the blistering stage. Avoid nylon, rubber or plastic footwear and rubber gloves as this type of eczema can be aggravated by heat and sweating.

12

TREATMENTS

Although eczema cannot be cured it can usually be controlled. One of the problems with eczema is that although the skin can look good on the surface, it may not be healed completely underneath. It can then start itching and get scratched and cracked and the whole cycle is repeated, so you do need to keep up the moisturising routine.

Eczema can also clear up spontaneously or seem totally under control. In either event, remember that you have a dry skin which must be moisturised at all times.

Bathing, moisturising and treating the skin is the daily routine for most people with eczema. Some people may find that water irritates their skin and they may need to curtail the frequency and duration of bath times.

Please note that the products mentioned in this chapter are just some of those currently available. This is not a recommendation that they are all suitable for everyone with eczema and it is not a fully comprehensive listing.

· *Bathing* ·

Most people with eczema benefit from daily baths *providing* that the water is not too hot, an emollient is added to the bath water and a soap-substitute is used. Never use bubble bath as it dries out the skin. Bathing can help replace the moisture that is lost from an eczematous skin and adding an emollient to the bath water helps lock that moisture into the skin. Here is a bath routine you might like to follow for yourself or for your child with eczema:

● Run a bath of *WARM* water. Please make sure it is not hot. Add one or two cupfuls of one of the bath oils listed below or, if you prefer, you can dissolve a tablespoon of emulsifying ointment in boiling water, mix with a fork and add it to the bath water.

● Spend about 20 minutes in the bath as this gives the skin time to absorb the oils. However, if there are very itchy, open wounds you will need to cut short this time.

● Take a lump of emulsifying ointment into your hands and gently massage it onto the skin as you would soap. Make sure that you cover the eczematous areas especially. Rinse off and then repeat if necessary. Try and encourage your child to join in the bath routine but never leave a child in the bath on his own and remember that he will be very slippery when coming out.

Pat the skin dry with a soft towel, leaving it slightly moist. Now is the time to apply the emollients and steroid creams or ointments if you are currently using them.

· *Bath oils and emulsifiers* ·

Oilatum Emollient (contains lanolin)
Aveeno Oilated
Balneum
Emulsiderm
Bath E45

You can use a soap-substitute instead of emulsifier to cleanse the skin. The following do not contain irritant alkaline or perfume:

Imuderm Body Wash
Wash E45
Emulave Bar

· *Moisturising and treating* ·

If topical steroids are in use apply them before the emollient. Whether you use a cream or an ointment is a question of personal choice. Ointments are greasy and give the best results on a dry skin. Creams are not greasy and therefore don't leave the skin feeling sticky. A good compromise would be to use an ointment at night and a cream during the day.

Always wash your hands before applying creams or ointments. Also make sure that containers are closed tightly straight after use. Eczematous skin can become infected if the contents of the container are contaminated. A pump dispenser is helpful in this respect.

If you have more than one eczematous person in the family, make sure each has their own supply of emollients to avoid cross-infection.

Apply thinly and smooth in. If the preparation you are using is thick, apply it in small dots on the parts of the body affected, working from the head to the toes. They will have melted and become more manageable by the time you come to gently smooth them in.

Although applying moisturisers straight from the bath is the most beneficial, you should use them at least twice a day.

REMEMBER: Don't stop the treatment as soon as the skin looks better. It can look good on the surface but it may not be healed thoroughly underneath.

· *Emollients* ·

Emollients are mixtures of water, waxes, fats and oils in varying proportions. Basically, they are moisturisers. When the surface of skin is damaged, it lets the moisture out which makes dry eczematous skin even more dry and stiff. This is when it can start to crack, and a dried-out skin can be very itchy. Applied regularly, emollients can provide a film of oil on the skin which prevents the loss of moisture from inside. This film can also act as a barrier against outside irritants.

Emollients are safe to use and rarely cause allergic reaction. But occasionally, products containing lanolin, which is a fat derived from sheep's wool, can have this effect. Finding out which products suit you is a matter of trial and error.

Emollient brands

Aquadrate
Aqueous Cream
Calmurid
Cream E45 (contains lanolin)
Diprobase
Eczederm
Emulsiderm
Emulsifying ointment
Hydromol cream
Keri Lotion (contains lanolin)

Lipobase
Neurtrogena body Oil
Nutraplus
Oilatum Cream
Probase 3
Sudocrem
Ultrabase
Unguentum Merk
Vaseline Dermacare
  cream

· *Topical steroids* ·

Steroids are a group of natural hormones produced by the body. Amongst other functions, they help the healing process. Artificially produced steroids aim to have the same effect. Topical steroids are the ones that you apply to the site of the problem and they are extremely useful in treating eczema. But they must be used with caution. Steroids should be applied in as small a quantity as possible once or twice a day and only on patches of affected skin. Once you have placed the steroid on the skin allow it to sink in before you apply moisturiser, otherwise you will dilute the strength and efficacy of the steroid.

Sometimes, if the skin is very inflamed, it is worth using a stronger steroid for a short period to bring the inflammation down and then continue treating with a mild topical steroid until you have the condition under control.

Steroids do not cure eczema but they can speed up the healing process. They can also reduce itchiness. But used indiscriminately they can cause side effects. Very heavy usage of potent topical steroids could, if used over a long period of time, restrict growth. You may find this extraordinary because the steroid is applied outside the body. But remember skin is permeable and the cream or ointment is able to penetrate the layers to where the eczema actually occurs. So some of it will get into the bloodstream. Tiny amounts in the bloodstream are not going to cause any deleterious effect. Larger amounts could cause a similar effect to steroids taken by mouth. In addition to affecting growth they can also cause thinning and reddening of skin and stretch marks.

One of the main difficulties in topical steroid treatment is getting the amount right. Using too little can render the treatment ineffectual and too much can cause side effects. The stronger the steroids the more cautious you will need to be in using them. You also need to take into consideration whereabouts on the body they are to be applied, and the person's body weight. The smaller the person, the lower the body weight and the more cautious you need to be about the amount of steroids used. You will need to use a lot less on a child than on an adult.

Fingertip dosing unit

Recently a guideline has been suggested to help eczema patients assess how much of the topical steroids constitutes a single application. This is known as the Fingertip Dosing Unit. *One unit is the amount of cream or ointment it takes to cover an adult finger from its tip to the crease of the next joint.* This is one strip of the ointment or cream as it comes out of the nozzle of an ordinary tube. Whether the amount you need to treat an area should be one unit or 14 units depends on which area of the body you are treating. The following doses are for an adult. A very young child will need one-quarter of the adult dose, a four-year-old will need a third.

- One hand needs 1 fingertip unit
- One foot needs 2 fingertip units

- One arm needs 3 fingertip units
- One leg needs 6 fingertip units
- Trunk (front and back) needs 14 fingertip units.

Topical steroids are made up of a base substance which can be an ointment or cream which carries the active drug. This cream or ointment dilutes the active ingredients and the above dose guidelines have been formulated with the diluted cream/ointment in mind.

Topical steroids are *not* for use on infected eczema or mild eczema. Infected eczema is described in Chapter 11.

I have grouped the steroids listed below in order of strength or potency: Group 1 being very high and Group 4 being low. Whether you use a cream, ointment or lotion is a question of choice, but ointment is generally preferred. Please note that this list is not fully comprehensive and is only intended as a guide and not a recommendation.

Group 1 – Very potent

Dermovate	*Nerisone Forte*
Dermovate NN	*Halciderm*

These are generally *not* suitable for young children. Older children may use them but for short periods in limited areas. *Never* use them on the face or eyelids and *never* without medical advice. Use a very thin smear applied with one fingertip on the affected area only once or twice a day at the most. If you are using this strength you should keep in regular contact with your doctor. Inform him or her if the eczema has not improved after a week of treatment and get in touch with the doctor immediately if the condition gets worse. To ensure that you are using the correct amount, ask the doctor how long the tube should last you.

Group 2 – Potent

Propaderm	*Nerisone*	*Locoid C*
Diprosone	*Topilar*	*Adcortyl*
Betnovate	*Synalar*	*Nystadermal*
Betnovate C	*Synalar N*	*Tri-Adcortyl*
Elocon	*Locoid*	

The same comments apply for this group as Group 1.

Group 3 – Moderately potent

Betnovate RD	Synalar 1:4	Alphaderm
Eumovate	Ultradil plain	Calmudrid HC
Stiedex LP	Haelan	

These can be used for longer periods and very occasionally on the face. You can see them on young children when the eczema is very severe but only for a short time. Use sparingly and only on eczematous skin, once or twice a day. Keep in touch with your doctor if you are using this potency.

Group 4 – Mildly potent

Synalar 1:10	Epifoam	Terra-cortril
Canestan HC	Fucidin H	Terra-Cortril nystatin
Daktacort	Hydrocortistab	Timodine
Econacort	Hydrocortisyl	Vioform
Efcortelan	Quinocort	hydrocortisone

These are generally safe for all age groups, but should only be used for short periods on the very young.

There are some preparations that contain more than one active constituent. These may include steroids to speed the healing process, antibiotics to suppress infection and fungicides to suppress fungal and yeast infections. Preparations can contain any combination of base or actives and doctors prescribe different combinations to suit different conditions.

· Systemic steroids ·

These are sometimes used for severe eczema. They are very effective but they have significant side effects. In children they restrict growth. In adults they cause softening of the bones which is the condition known as osteoporosis. These are the two most important side effects, but there are others. For these reasons they are usually only used for short periods. They can be taken orally in the form of liquid or tablets, or by injection.

· Bandaging ·

These can be used to prevent scratching, protect the affected area or to allow medication to be well absorbed.

Crêpe bandages are good for protection but tubular ones are easier to use. You can get the latter in different sizes for different parts of the body.

Medicated bandages are very useful for treating severe eczema, particularly when the skin has become thick and leathery. They are used very effectively to treat varicose eczema. Many people find these bandages, soaked in ichthopaste, which combines zinc oxide with ichthammol, very soothing. Other pastes used are *Coltapaste* (zinc paste and coal tar) and *Cortacream* (1 percent hydrocortisone). The bandages have a cooling effect, relieve irritation and itchiness and speed up healing. They can be wet and very messy so you will need to cover these bandages with a dry bandage and the best one for this is called *Coban*, which you can get from chemists or hospital pharmacies.

· *Occlusion* ·

This method is used to achieve maximum absorption of medication – usually potent topical steroids. First the medication is applied and a tubular bandage is placed over it. Then comes the plastic or polythene film which is put on top of the bandage and firmly held in place by some form of sticky tape. This plastic occlusion greatly accelerates the rate at which the medication is absorbed through the skin and into the body. Steroids used this way get into the blood stream in much larger quantities than in the normal way.

· *Antihistamines* ·

Oral antihistamines can be very useful in treating eczema. They do not cure the condition but they do cut down on scratching. There is no evidence that taking large doses of antihistamines over a long period of time will make you addicted to them. (There are also other ways of trying to control the itch, one is the behavioural technique described later on in this chapter. Hypnotherapy can also be effective, as described in Chapter 14.)

An effect of antihistamines is that they make you sleepy and you cannot switch to the non-sedative kind because these do not seem to work for eczema. So driving could be a problem. Antihistamines are best taken at night, at least an hour before you go to bed to try and avoid the hangover effect.

Remember that some antihistamines can make your skin sensitive to sunlight, so check with your doctor if the one you are on has this effect. Also remember that antihistamine *creams* should not be used by people with eczema as they can cause an allergic reaction.

· *Ultraviolet therapy* ·

Since many people with atopic eczema find the condition improves in the sunlight, treatment with artificial sunlight sources has been tried over the years. This treatment, which is available in some dermatology clinics, is usually reserved for adult patients with severe atopic eczema who have not responded to other more traditional treatments. The link between ultraviolet rays and cancer is one of the reasons why ultraviolet therapy is not used generally for the treatment of eczema. It is also expensive to administer and inconvenient for the patient who has to attend the hospital two or three times a week. This treatment is known as UVB treatment which stands for Ultraviolet B.

PUVA treatment combines the use of a *psoralen* drug (hence the P) with ultraviolet light A. Patients are given the drug either topically or orally some hours before exposure to ultraviolet light. PUVA treatment is more commonly used for psoriasis than eczema.

· *Cyclosporin* ·

This is a new drug treatment available for some people with severe atopic eczema. Cyclosporin is used in the main for transplant patients as it suppresses the rejection of transplanted organs. It has also been found to be very useful in treating eczema.

According to Dr Berth-Jones, Senior Registrar in Dermatology at the Leicester Royal Infirmary, Cyclosporin works by dampening down strong allergic and immune reactions. Writing in the National Eczema Society's newsletter, *Exchange*, Dr Berth-Jones says:

Although the cause of atopic eczema is not fully understood, it is clear that immunological reactions are occurring in the skin and these are controlled by white blood cells (lymphocytes) which enter the skin from the blood. Cyclosporin has numerous actions on the immune system which tend to dampen down strong allergic and immune reactions. The most important effect is probably the inhibition of production by lymphocytes of chemicals called *cytokines*. Cytokines act as messengers to 'switch on' other lymphocytes and they are essential for immunological and allergic reactions to build up strength.

The net result is that some nine out of ten people with eczema find that the condition greatly improves when taking Cyclosporin. Of course it would be wonderful if it was all good news but any drug that suppresses the immune system should not be taken lightly and Cyclosporin is no different.

People who have any serious infections, or may be suffering from cancer or who have had cancer in the past are not advised to take this drug. People who have a history of kidney disease, liver disease, high blood pressure, diabetes or high blood cholesterol may not be prescribed Cyclosporin. Pregnant women will also not be prescribed this drug.

Another point to bear in mind is that Cyclosporin does not *cure* eczema. While you are taking it the eczema gets better but once you come off the treatment the condition tends to re-appear.

Since it is important to be monitored when taking this drug, it is usually prescribed by dermatologists and not, as a rule, by G.P.s.

Obviously someone with mild eczema would not take this drug as the disadvantages would outweigh the benefits. But for someone with severe eczema it is worth considering. As Dr Berth-Jones says:

> The drug is best reserved for patients whose lives are being severely disrupted by the disease. The quality of patients' lives improves considerably. They feel less embarrassed by their eczema, they are less distracted from their work by soreness and itching, they can enjoy their leisure time more effectively and they can sleep better at night.

· *Behavioural approach* ·

One method of tackling chronic eczema which includes no oral drugs and has no side effects is being pioneered at the Daniel Turner Skin Clinic at London's Chelsea and Westminster Hospital. The key to this technique is to try and take the scratching out of the condition and by doing so turn it into an illness that may appear from time to time but never stays for longer than a few days.

Writing in *Exchange*, Dr Christopher Bridgett, Consultant Psychiatrist at the Daniel Turner Skin Clinic says:

> Without scratching, chronic eczema cannot exist. Dry skin and acute eczema will respond quickly to the proper use of emollients and topical steroids. If scratching becomes established, then so does chronic eczema, and topical treatment with emollients and steroids fails to cure the condition.

The dermatological treatment offered at this skin clinic is rather different to that elsewhere. First comes the 'assessment' – a history of the condition and looking at the record of relapses, as well as an analysis of the patient's scratching behaviour. No one scratches all the time, so a pattern usually emerges. How you scratch and what effect this has on your family is also considered. The therapist uses the individual pattern to draw-up a tailor-made programme of treatment.

Between the first and second visits to the clinic patients are asked to keep a record of their scratching 'registration'. The theory is that much scratching takes place at an unconscious level. Whether you have eczema or not, much of the time you are scratching, you are doing so without being aware of it. 'Registration' means becoming aware of scratching. Treatment continues at the second visit with an explanation of the role of emollients and topical steroids in eczema so that you know how to get the best out of these treatments. Then the scratch is tackled. This is known as 'habit reversal' – you learn to replace the scratching with something that doesn't damage the skin. For the first 30 seconds of the impulse to scratch you close your fist and fix the joints of the upper limbs. If after this you still want to scratch you pinch the area of skin that you would otherwise scratch. You do this until the need to scratch goes away. Gradually you learn to respond to the itch in a way that doesn't damage your skin.

Follow-up treatments are designed to help patients arrive at a programme that will work for them. Apparently children respond to a similar technique very well. The treatment lasts a few weeks.

The Consultant Dermatologist in charge of this treatment at the Daniel Turner Clinic is Dr Richard Staughton. If you are interested in getting treatment you will need a referral from your G.P.

· *Products for people with eczema* ·

Shampoos useful for treating seborrhoeic eczema

Baltar (2 years and over)   Gelcotar Liquid
Betadine   Genisol
Ceanel   Ionil T
Cetavlon   Polytar
Clinitar   Synogist
Cradocap (children only)   T-Gel

Shampoos you can use when the condition is under control

Neutrogena Mild Shampoo   Simple

Sunscreens that suit people with eczema

Almay Sun Bloc Cream 15
Coppertone Supershade 15
Roc Total Sunblock

Sun E45
Soltan 20 (UVA)
Uvistat

13

DOCTORS, SPECIALISTS AND SKIN TESTS

· *Doctors* ·

My daughter was 18 months old when her eczema became very severe. I made repeated visits to my G.P., who never examined her and said he would not alter her treatment in any way. I had a tube of a strong steroid cream. I had not heard of emollients and obviously neither had my G.P.! I went privately to see a dermatologist, who very soon admitted my daughter to hospital, having transferred her back to the NHS. She was prescribed oral steroids to get an improvement in her by then chronic eczema. I have now changed my G.P. to a much more sympathetic one. I can only recommend that anyone experiencing similar problems should do the same.

The above is an excerpt from a letter which appeared in the National Eczema Society's magazine *Exchange*. People are not always happy about the service they get from their doctor and there are three common grumbles. Firstly, it is generally felt that doctors don't take the condition seriously enough; secondly, the treatments are not fully explained and thirdly, some G.P.s are reluctant to refer their patients to specialists.

Of course the doctor should be taking your skin condition seriously. Along with the diagnosis, the doctor should help you look at some of the environmental situations and personal circumstances that could be triggering or aggravating the condition. Questions about your home, pets, diet, family, work – even make-up – can point a finger at why the eczema has suddenly appeared or become worse.

Once the doctor has prescribed treatment, he or she should explain it thoroughly to you. It is very important that you know the difference between the emollients and steroid creams and the different roles that they play. Take a notebook and jot down the names of the creams the doctor is prescribing, what they do and how often you should use them. If you've been prescribed steroid creams ask how long you are supposed to be using them and also ask about side effects.

Never get a steroid preparation on repeat prescription. The

doctor should examine your skin to make sure there is no damage occurring and to check that skin is not infected.

Very occasionally, patients find that the pharmacist looks at the prescription and says: "This is much too potent a steroid, you shouldn't be using it on your face/baby etc." Don't just not use it, or use a little bit and stop. Contact your doctor and tell him what the pharmacist has said and explain that you are worried. The doctor may have prescribed this strong steroid for a short while to stop the eczema in its tracks, or stop a chronic cycle. If you are worried – check it out. You can always contact the National Eczema Society who run a steroid information line in the afternoon.

If you have carried out your doctor's prescribed treatment to the best of your ability and the eczema still hasn't cleared and it is affecting your life, you have every right to ask to be referred to a specialist.

Changing doctors

If you are not happy with your doctor it is really very easy to change. Make an appointment with a possible new doctor and say that eczema is a particular concern of yours and you were wondering what he or she feels about eczema patients and what were the sort of treatments he or she believes are helpful to the condition. Some doctors have a real problem with patients with chronic illness like eczema. They get very frustrated with patients they cannot cure. Others have a more realistic understanding of the problem.

When you have found a doctor that you want to move to, make sure that the practice is willing to take you on. If they are, you must now write to your current doctors' practice and tell them that you are moving and where you are moving to. This is so that your medical records are sent to the new practice. You don't have to give the out-going doctor any reasons for your move. You will then need to wait a couple of weeks for your medical records to reach their new destination.

If you would like any more information on changing doctors you can ring the Regional Health Information Service on 0800 665544. This is a national number which you ring and are automatically put through to your region.

· *Specialists* ·

There are benefits in being referred to a dermatologist. A dermatologist is in a better position to determine how severe a patient's eczema is than is a G.P. and will be able to check for infection more quickly. Since the dermatologist has specialised in treating skin conditions, he or she will have a more up-to-date knowledge of the new treatments on offer. This will include traditional treatments in the shape of pills, potions, creams and bandaging as well as some of the alternatives like Chinese herbal medicine. A dermatologist may be able to assess the suitability of an alternative therapy and be able to prescribe it. The dermatologist can also assess whether or not any of the tests sometimes used for eczema and explained below are going to be of use to your particular condition.

However, lack of time is a real problem in dermatology clinics in the U.K. and many eczema patients come away from them feeling dissatisfied. Most clinics are run on the basis of between five and eight minutes per patient and this is not usually long enough to treat eczema patients.

The dermatologist will probably give you more time than this but go prepared for brevity. Make a note of the questions you want to ask but don't take a long list. Focus on the issues that your G.P. cannot help you with. But remember that you have every right to see a specialist. It is not a free service but paid for out of *your* taxes!

· *Allergy tests* ·

As explained in Chapter 2 atopic people tend to make larger than usual amounts of antibodies called *immunoglobin E* (*IgE*) which is there to help defend the body against substances that it is allergic to. Some of the tests carried out are done to measure the amount of *IgE* the body produces when it comes into contact with a known allergen. This is thought to give some indication as to whether or not the person is allergic to that substance. The two most commonly used tests are the Skin Prick Test and the RAST test (short for Radio-AllergoSorbent Test). Neither are used widely for atopic eczema because it is difficult to obtain highly accurate results, and as these people can be allergic to such a variety of different things, identifying one or two may be very little help. Patch testing, which is carried out for allergic contact eczema, seems to be a more reliable and helpful exercise.

Skin prick test

For this test a solution is made up which contains a small amount of a possible allergy-creating substance such as cat dander, pollen, dust or a food product. This is introduced into the skin by gently pricking it with a sterile needle and dropping the solution into the slightly 'opened' area. If you are allergic to the substance, there will be a reaction in the shape of a slightly raised lump or weal about fifteen minutes later.

RAST test

A small amount of blood is taken from one of the patient's veins to measure the level of *immunoglobin E* in the blood. There are certain types of *IgE* in the blood which defend the body against specific allergens such as pollens, cat dander and some foods. This test can confirm that you are atopic, but positive results do not necessarily indicate that the eczema is caused by the substance tested.

Patch tests

This is a very useful test for anyone who has allergic contact dermatitis. If you have eczema on your hands or feet ask your doctor to refer you to a dermatology clinic where it can be carried out. The dermatologist will ask for details of your skin problems together with information about the kind of materials you handle at work or use regularly at home or in the course of a hobby or social activity. All this is done to try and determine what possible substance or substances may be causing the reaction. You should add to this any other substances that you suspect you could be sensitive to. For those with eczema on the feet for instance, chromate could be a possible allergen. Nickel, rubber and other chemicals are known to produce sensitivity in some people.

A diluted version of each possible allergen is then put on different areas of a piece of filter paper and this is applied to an unaffected area of your body, usually the back. The paper is stuck on with some adhesive tape and left in place for 48 hours. The patch is then removed and the skin is examined. You may then be asked to return 48 hours after that when the skin is examined again. It is very important to return for this check. If the skin is itchy, red and swollen in some places, the dermatologist will check what was on these particular areas of filter paper to determine what it is you are allergic to. You should then try and avoid coming into contact with the substances that cause the problem. Although patch testing sounds simple you shouldn't try to do it yourself. It really is a specialist's job!

Skin biopsy

This is usually done by a dermatologist to get an accurate diagnosis of the type of eczema you have. It entails removing a small piece of skin and is usually done under a local anaesthetic. You may need one or two stitches but the whole procedure is very quick.

PSYCHOLOGICAL INPUT

There are psychological factors present in most illnesses as the mind is the most powerful and volatile part of our make-up, and I don't believe that you can look at a chronic condition like eczema without examining the psychological input.

Many people working in the psychotherapeutic fields say that eczema is not only a disease of the skin but also an outlet for a person's emotions. During the course of our lives we inevitably experience emotional conflict, upset or even trauma that we cannot adequately deal with. There may be a few people who are able to deal with emotional issues in a totally pragmatic and uninvolved way. Most of us cannot do this, at least not every time, and the conflict or unhappiness stays with us in the form of unfinished business which may then express itself in the shape of migraine, colitis, asthma, psoriasis, eczema and other illnesses.

This way of dealing with emotional issues can start at a very young age. Even a baby can pick up feelings of anxiety, tenseness and unhappiness that his parents may be experiencing. The baby may cry a lot or he may become itchy and eczematous. And once this response has been triggered it is likely to repeat itself time and time again. So as a young child and then as an adult, stress, conflict or trauma can trigger the eczema.

If you are the parents of a child with eczema please don't add guilt to the load you may already be carrying. There is no way that you can stop yourself from having feelings. Repressed feelings or emotions find an outlet one way or another. And in as much as you cannot stop feeling, you cannot stop your children from picking up feelings and expressing them in their own way. I too have a child who had eczema very severely as a youngster, so what I hope I am doing here is sharing an experience.

Just because we cannot stop something doesn't mean that we cannot deal with it. You may not be able to prevent yourself from having emotions but you can learn to deal with them in a manner that is less harmful. One way to do that is to learn to express feeling verbally. If, as a person with eczema, you can say: "I found this hurtful because . . .", "I don't like what you said because . . .", and get into the habit of off-loading your emotions in this way, you might find that you stop expressing them through your skin. The more up-front you can get with your emotions the less likely you are to be locked into the conditioned response of stress/eczema. If as a parent of a child with eczema you can help him or her, or even the whole family, to get into the habit of recognising their feelings and talking about them, you could do a lot for the family's general health, let alone a particular skin condition.

Most people are likely to agree that if you have had eczema over a long period of time it may have a bearing on your personality, particularly if you have not been able to talk about the condition in a relaxed and open way.

Take the case of 12-year-old Tessa (not her real name) whose eczema is consistently severe, but when it flares it is so sore that she daren't move because the skin stretches and cracks and, needless to say, is extremely painful. Yet the teachers at school do not seem to have noticed her distress because they do not give her enough time to apply her creams and she daren't ask them for fear of being thought different.

She is sometimes on oral steroids and extremely worried about the effect they may be having on her, yet no one has talked to her about this and she says that no one talks to her about her skin. She goes into hospital regularly and at one time, when she was about 10 years old, she was actually tied down to stop her from scratching. This 'preventative' treatment stopped when her mother went in and threw a 'wobbly' at the staff. This happened in modern times and in a British hospital!

Fortunately, tying people down to stop them from scratching is not widely practised, but what is widespread is the experience of no one talking about the condition. Time and time again people with eczema have reported that no one talks to them about their skin.

Suppose, for instance, you were teased at school, it is very likely that you learned to cover up the hurt you felt. You learned not to give your tormentors any satisfaction and to hide how you felt, possibly not only from them, but from yourself as well. We learn, quite early on, to block off painful feelings.

Although you may have forgotten all about the teasing and harassment now, this learned behaviour may well have become part of your personality, and you may have got into the habit of not recognising pain or conflict for what it is. Somewhere in your subconscious is the message: "This is painful or stressful and I cannot handle it, so let's forget about it." But stresses, anxieties and conflicts do not go away just because you are not thinking about them; they come out in another way and for you that way could be eczema.

A condition like eczema can change a person's outlook on life. Most of us, particularly when we are young, do not believe that anything bad can happen to us. It can happen to the person down the road but somehow we feel we have some kind of special protection from the bad things. When you've been the one who has had to put up with a condition that sets you apart from other people and makes you feel different, it is possible that instead of feeling 'protected' from life's disasters, you will feel singled out to be the recipient of some of the bad things in life. These feelings need to be discussed and understood for what they are and then, hopefully, discarded forever.

Starting to talk about your feelings, if this has never been your way, is not easy. If you have spent a lifetime keeping your feelings under wraps, you are unlikely to turn into a person who bends the ears of his friends and neighbours on a daily basis. It may be very important to you to remain a private person. The thought of sharing your feelings with the world at large may seem very threatening. Counselling and psychotherapy exist for people who want to get in touch with their feelings but want to do so in a private way.

I have also included a short description of hypnotherapy in this chapter as that also focuses on the patient's mind to help alleviate the condition.

· *Counselling* ·

A counsellor's job is to look at the here and now and examine current patterns of behaviour. He or she will encourage you to talk freely without fear of being judged or criticised in any way. But the counsellor is also trained to try and find out 'where you are coming from' and relate current feelings and behaviour to experiences that have happened in the past. He or she will delve a little into childhood and family background to try and get a clearer picture of you as a person. Over a period of time, this kind of examination of why you do the things you do can help you see yourself in a new light and help you to understand more about your feelings and motivations.

What counselling can also do is to help rid you of some of your emotional ghosts. To carry on the theme of teasing, for instance, talking to a counsellor about it and re-living it perhaps many years on, may be painful, but once you've brought the episode back up, re-lived it and looked at it without the same vulnerabilities, you may then be able to walk away from it. These kinds of talking treatments are good at helping you dispose of unwanted and destructive emotional luggage. They are also very useful in current emotional situations. If you are going through a bad patch or unhappy period of your life, talking to a counsellor can help you express your anger and hurt and in so doing, ease the pain. Counselling is not supposed to be a destructive process – quite the contrary. The aim of peeling back the layers and helping you to know more about yourself is that it should strengthen you, give you more personal power and enable you to feel good about yourself.

With counselling all this takes place at a conscious level. Psychotherapy digs a bit deeper.

· *Psychotherapy* ·

With psychotherapy the useful work takes place in the unconscious. It looks at your internal as well as external world. Our external world involves our day-to-day activities and how we react to them. Our internal world is made up of memories, thoughts, dreams and fantasies that we are aware of as well as the desires, fears and fantasies that we are not conscious of. It is getting to know and understanding this internal world that is the art of psychotherapy. A skilled psychotherapist can unlock many doors and enable you to understand yourself better and express your feelings in a more productive and less damaging way.

Since psychotherapy goes deeper into the person's psyche it is usually a much more long-term treatment than counselling. First of all a relationship of trust needs to build up between client and psychotherapist and this of course takes time.

There are special techniques used in psychotherapy to help the therapist unlock the patient's unconscious. Dream interpretation is one such technique. When a person is dreaming they are open to feelings and moods that may be blocked when they are awake. Also when we dream we communicate more in visual images than words and it is the therapist's job to interpret these visual images which may throw light on a person's deeply hidden fears, longings or emotional pain.

There are many other techniques that psychotherapists can use to get into their clients' subconscious which bit by bit can put you in touch with past experiences and current motivations.

· *Hypnotherapy* ·

In this form of therapy the aim is to shift the patient's attention from external to internal awareness. It may sound complex but apparently there are many techniques for achieving this and it does not take very long.

With hypnotherapy much of the work goes on in the patient's subconscious mind. The patient is put into a trance state which is similar to day dreaming or the slowing down, drifting feeling before you drop off to sleep.

When in the hypnotic state, people tend to be much more receptive to therapy in the form of suggestions and imagery, as the left side of the brain, which is in charge of analytical and logical thought, shuts off. The therapist can communicate with the patient's subconscious mind without the blocks and defences that would usually exist. Most patients remember almost everything that has happened while in a trance state.

With eczema patients the therapist will explore possible underlying problems that may be causing the condition. This may include finding out about the patient's lifestyle, investigating causes of stress and looking at the level of confidence and self-esteem in the patient. Therapy may then focus on these possible problems, as well as dealing directly with alleviation of eczema symptoms such as itching or burning.

Many therapists also employ visualisation techniques with their patients. For example, a patient may be asked to visualise in their mind that they are somewhere peaceful, such as lying on a raft, with each gentle sway of the raft allowing them to feel more relaxed. For people who are not good at seeing visual imagery in their minds, they can use their other senses to imagine being in such a place.

This process can be made even more enjoyable by positive and soothing self-talk, such as telling yourself for example: "I am feeling calm," "I am in control" or "My body is feeling relaxed." The process of visualisation, which involves full participation of the patient's conscious mind, can often naturally lead to a hypnotic state where conscious participation is greatly lessened.

Elaine Sheehan is a hypnotherapist who has qualified in applied psychology. She is also a trainer and lecturer with British Hypnosis Research. She says:

> Before I teach a patient self-hypnosis I will usually first of all work on any possible underlying problems which may be contributing to feelings of stress and anxiety, such as negative thinking patterns, poor self-image and lack of confidence . . . I get them used to the process and able to identify when they are in this special relaxed state. Once they have experienced that a few times I teach them self-hypnosis . . . In a state of hypnosis the patient can become deeply relaxed. The aim is not only to achieve positive feelings at the time, but to carry these feelings over into the future through the use of post-hypnotic suggestions which can make you a more relaxed person in general . . . You are giving yourself suggestions to be a certain way. You are telling your mind what you want for yourself rather than accepting whatever comes along. You may not be in control of life's circumstances and events, but you can be in control of how you choose to respond to them.

Therapists vary in the number of sessions they consider will effectively treat eczema, but it is not a long-term therapy. As a rule of thumb you can reckon on anything between two and six sessions.

Anyone experiencing eczema in the genital area may like to consider this therapy. This part of the body can be difficult to treat in an external way, so this treatment may well be worth a try.

Michael Joseph who is the president of the Association of Clinical Hypnotherapists says that patients, whether adult or child, are first put into a light trance to discover the underlying causes and then taught self-hypnosis to teach them to relax. They may also be given post-hypnotic suggestions to relieve their symptoms.

He says:

> We hypnotise the patient and suggest, for instance, that any affected area of their skin will become much cooler. With some people you can actually give direct suggestions that the eczema clears and sometimes it does.
>
> If you have not dealt with the underlying causes it will usually return. Sometimes even if you have dealt with the underlying causes the skin rash will remain as a conditioned reflex and then you can remove it by direct suggestion.

Treatment for eczema is usually short – Mr Joseph says he has never seen a person with eczema more than twice. Although visualisation is explained to patients, Mr Joseph believes that patients can learn to do this by themselves once they have been taught self-hypnosis, avoiding costly visits to the therapist.

> Eczema often recurs later on in an individual's life when they are under pressure again, [says Mr Joseph]. Once the nervous system learns to react to stressful situations with a rash, when anything happens that reminds the brain of the eczema, it (the brain) will bring it on again. It's a conditioned reflex and I have never been able to eradicate the eczema completely, if I'm honest. I have had people who have come back years later saying it has suddenly started again. We try again and then I don't see them for another few years.

Both the Association of Clinical Hypnosis and British Hypnosis Research have members nationwide. BHR publishes a register of their practitioners listing the particular problems they specialise in. Addresses are in Chapter 17.

· JIM ·

I have had eczema since I was two years old. I am now 21 and still have it. I had never spoken to anyone about my eczema until recently, but as I found myself talking to someone who had time to listen, I felt a tiny amount of my lifelong burden escape its grasp.

The eczema was on my face, arms and legs as well as the joints. It was very noticeable. Now and again you feel so short of confidence that you don't show your face anywhere. You try and keep yourself to yourself. When you're really bad you don't want to face anything.

I was never in the popular end of the class. I was generally very shy due to my skin. But in the Sixth Form I started to fight back and try and be noticed instead of hiding at the back of the class. I became very loud and blasé to cover up the shyness. I had a good time but deep down, emotionally, I think I was still hiding.

I am trying to analyse where my complexes about doing things and meeting people come from. I find meeting people and feeling confident with people very hard.

Between the ages of five and 15 you accept it. You think it's just life and you don't analyse it. You take it for granted and think that that's the way it is. But when you get older you see that other people don't hold back and aren't shy. As soon as I started art college I started to get into philosophy and stuff like that and I started to question things about myself. It's been non-stop thinking ever since and it's been quite complicated.

There are times when I wake up in the morning and get out of bed and the minute my skin hits the air it gets really sore. The feeling of going to bed and knowing that the next morning your skin is going to be so sore can be very hard to handle. Especially if it happens over a long period of time.

It's only in the past few years that the eczema has really started to come on my face. Even when it's not visible I feel vulnerable even though I may not look bad. It feels very sore. I get very dry lips and it doesn't half hurt to laugh or even sneeze. The eyes are the worst because they very easily get sore even when the skin is good. All I have to do is rub them a couple of times when it is raining – the rain drops make them sore.

When I went to school I'd have to walk about half an hour to the bus stop every morning. I'd get a horrible flush on my face and it felt like it was on fire. It was a bit like having acid on your face, it was so sore. It was something I couldn't control.

Most people seem to have excellent complexions and you tend to feel that because you look different, you are different. It makes you feel twice as bad when you look in the mirror and see this blotch. For a while I had a huge sore ring around my mouth. I used to get a lot of teasing for that.

I'm depressed a lot of the time, but I try not to let it get me down. I sometimes feel incredible mental stress but I have built a strong personality around myself to compensate for my shyness. I go through incredible pain which I keep to myself. Sometimes I hurt so bad I feel like screaming "I'm in pain" but I usually end up keeping the feeling to myself or just writing it down.

You can treat the eczema indefinitely but the emotional problems are always going to be there and they are going to continue to grow. It's a vicious circle: you feel tense and that makes your skin worse and you scratch – you can't resist the scratching.

I didn't meet another person with eczema until last year when I joined the National Eczema Society. I am now writing to about five or six. Hearing from people who have had exactly the same experiences is really helping. I've always found talking to people who don't have it like talking to a brick wall. You can go so far but you have got to understand you can't go further than that. I've tried so many times.

Having eczema has made me a different kind of person. A lot of people I am writing to mention how sensitive and caring they are. Apart from the way I have been brought up in the family, having eczema has been instrumental in making me the sort of person I am. Most of the time I wish I'd never had it but at other times I feel grateful. I see life in a completely different way. I've got so much will to do something with my life.

· TARA ·
(not her real name)

In my family background I always felt I was the black sheep that couldn't keep up with the rest of the family. I felt different from them because I had this skin problem. I was always so conscious of the feeling that I wasn't good enough. I was different because of my skin. I almost felt that I wasn't a member of the human race. I belonged somewhere a bit different and somehow I had got into the wrong species. So there was always a struggle – rather than say anything, I was struggling to keep up and conform.

At boarding school I felt very different to everybody else. Nobody else had eczema there. At the time I was seeing a homoeopathic specialist and he prescribed a cream that was smelly and horrible. I used to get called "smelly". The kids were horrible. I was 12 years old at the time. I boarded for two years and the first year I was in a huge dormitory with 24 people. I was very conscious of scratching at night and keeping others awake.

I went through a stage when I was in my late teens and early twenties when the eczema hardly affected my life at all apart from the odd flare-ups. It was quite a happy time. I had met somebody who I had fallen in love with. He was a very popular chap. He had a lot of friends and he introduced me to them. As his partner I found that I was very popular too. When we went out we were the centre of attention. We were the people who kept the party going. It made me feel great. I thought at last I don't have to be struggling to be somebody else, I am perfectly okay in my own right. That lasted for about five years. Then we split up. When I was going out with this chap my skin problem was still there but it wasn't running my life. I seemed to be able to do most things, whereas now it is running my life. Now I really have to lead my life around it.

Pregnancy was my turning point. After my baby was born I had marriage problems and my skin got worse and worse. Many times I can remember being absolutely suicidal with it. I really didn't know what to do with myself. It flared up all over my body which I hadn't experienced before, although fortunately it has never showed very much in my face. I've always been very grateful for that.

My husband was dreadful. It was mental cruelty in actual fact and it was similar to what I experienced with my family as a child. I realise now that subconsciously you actually attract people who keep you in the position that you've been used to. He was always putting me down. The annoying thing was that he was not like that at all before we were married. I didn't see a hint of it beforehand.

I am sure my emotional and psychological state has a big influence on my eczema. I've had counselling and I've also looked into Transactional Analysis and I'm actually taking a course on that now. I think that's why I'm a lot better this year. It's the TA and counselling that has made my life fit together. Before it was a total confused mess and nothing seemed to fit anywhere. Reading up on TA I could understand it all. It fitted in.

Having eczema has made me a different kind of person because of feeling different to everybody else from childhood onwards. It makes me feel as if I am a wimp in some way. People don't understand when you can't go to certain places. A lot of people cannot understand the allergy to cats and dogs. Dog lovers and cat lovers think that there's something completely wrong with you. They cannot acknowledge that you have an allergy – they think you don't like dogs. That kind of thing gets to you.

I think with eczema treatment the mental side of it is very much overlooked. Nobody seems to talk about it. I always felt that I was making a mountain out of a molehill. I'm still not buzzing over with confidence but I'm much better and that has been achieved through the counselling and the Transactional Analysis.

Anyone who would like to know more about Transactional Analysis, may like to contact The Institute of Transactional Analysis. The address can be found in Chapter 17.

ALTERNATIVE THERAPIES

There are a growing number of alternative or complementary treatments available in Britain. For a person with eczema who has tried traditional forms of medicine with no lasting success, looking into the possibilities of alternative therapies can be a positive move.

There are so many different treatments on offer that it is difficult to know which one to choose. One way is by personal recommendation. If a friend tells you that his or her eczema has improved with a particular therapy, regard it as one that is worth considering. But don't be disappointed if it doesn't work for you. As with creams and pills and other forms of orthodox medicine, what works for one doesn't necessarily do anything for another.

Another yardstick is your own feelings about any particular therapy. You need to have some feeling of belief in a particular therapy to be able to give it a serious try.

As with other forms of treatment, it is very important to go to a qualified practitioner. There are no laws governing complementary medicine in Britain at present so anyone can set up in practice. However, therapists tend to belong to an appropriate professional body and these usually require their members to have passed examinations and reached the required standard. So unless you are personally recommended to see a particular doctor or therapist contact the relevant professional body and ask them to recommend one in your area. Also remember that most complementary medicine is not available on the National Health, so you should find out the likely cost before embarking on any treatment.

The following short descriptions should give you an idea of the philosophy and methods behind just a few of the more popular complementary therapies on offer. Appropriate addresses appear in Chapter 17.

· *Acupuncture* ·

The term 'acupuncture' means 'needle piercing'. In China, where this treatment is practised widely, it is called *Chen chiu*, which means 'needle moxa'. *Moxa* is a dried herb which is burned in small cones on the skin, or on the handle of the needle, to generate a gentle heat. This method is known as *moxibustion*. Both these methods can be used during the course of acupuncture treatment.

Since the needles are so fine, there is no discomfort during the treatment but patients may feel a slight tingling. The needles may be left in for 20 minutes to half an hour, or they may be withdrawn immediately. The moxa is burned on, or held near to the point and removed when the patient feels that it is becoming too hot. This process is repeated several times.

Children or adults who have a fear of needles are usually given another form of treatment. This includes massage and tapping or pressure with a rounded probe. Alternatively they may receive electro-acupuncture and laser treatments in which the acupuncture points are stimulated either by a low frequency electrical current, applied direct with a probe, or with finely tuned laser beams. Gentle electrical stimuli may also be applied through the needles, giving a sensation of tingling or buzzing.

Acupuncture is part of a system of medicine that has been practised in China for several thousand years. More recently it has become widespread worldwide and research has taken place into its efficacy. One discovery has been that stimulation of acupuncture points induces the release by the brain of pain-relieving morphine-like substances known as *endorphins*. This may explain why acupuncture has been used so successfully as an alternative to anaesthetics in surgery.

Acupuncture is based on the principle that our health depends on the balanced functioning of the body's motivating energy. Known as *Chi*, this energy flows throughout the body but is concentrated in channels beneath the skin. These channels are called meridians and along them are the points by which the acupuncturist regulates the energy flow and bodily health.

The treatment aims to restore the harmony between the equal and opposite qualities of chi, the *yang* and the *yin*. Yang energy is aggressive. Yin energy is receptive. A dominance of yang energy in the body is thought to be experienced in the form of acute pain, headache, inflammation, spasms and high blood pressure. An excess of yin can be felt as dull aches and pains, chilliness, fluid retention, discharges and fatigue.

Practitioners of acupuncture aim to discover the nature of the disharmony in the body. They do this by careful questioning and observation: they will examine the patient's tongue for its structure, colour and coating and feel the pulses for their quality and strength. Once the cause of the problem has been diagnosed, the acupuncturist will select the points and the appropriate method of treatment.

Some G.P.s practise acupuncture in their surgeries. Others will be able to recommend a qualified practitioner. If you don't want to go through your G.P., you can find a qualified practitioner through the professional societies. Since needles are involved in the treatment, the big question is going to be about hepatitis and AIDS. Members of these professional bodies have to use needle sterilisation techniques approved by the Department of Health. These are considered to be effective against the hepatitis and AIDS viruses. Many practitioners use disposable needles.

· *Chinese herbal treatment* ·

This treatment has been found to be successful in treating some people with severe, atopic eczema. A few years ago the National Eczema Society and several leading dermatologists began to hear that some patients with eczema were being treated successfully with Chinese herbal medicine by Dr Ding Hui Luo in London. Together with other interested parties, the NES helped fund trials of this treatment and these were carried out with adults at the Royal Free Hospital in London under the direction of Dr Malcolm Rustin and with children at The Hospital for Sick Children, Great Ormond Street, London, under the direction of Dr David Atherton.

Normally, Chinese herbal medicine is prescribed on a personal basis. The herbal mix differs from patient to patient and the aim is to find a particular brew that will suit the particular individual and restore his or her body to health. However, for the purposes of the trial Dr Luo was asked to devise a standardised formulation that could be used by everybody participating in the study.

The reason for this was so that the herbs used could be checked for quality and also for toxicity to ensure, for example, that poisonous substances like mercury and arsenic were not used. The herbs were finely ground and put into sachets which resembled tea bags. These were brewed and consumed while still warm and apparently they tasted revolting.

The patients who took part in the study were specifically selected. They all had extensive eczema that had not responded to conventional treatment including steroids, but although the eczema was severe, it was not obviously infected and nor was it weepy.

Writing about the trials with children in his book: *Eczema in Children – The Facts*, Dr David Atherton explains that the trials included the real treatment which contained a mixture of parts of 10 different plants, all in common use as medicines in China, as well as a *placebo* which was a mixture of inert plant materials that looked and smelt similar to the real treatment but had no known benefit in atopic eczema.

Dr Atherton says:

We used a trial design known as 'cross-over', which means that every child would receive both the real treatment and the placebo treatment, each for eight successive weeks, with an intervening four-week period in which the effect of the first treatment would be 'washed out'. The order of the treatments was decided in a random way, that was only known to a third party, not to the doctors involved in the trial nor to the children or their parents. The children attended the clinic every four weeks throughout the five-month period.

All the children had blood checks to make sure that their bone marrow, kidneys and liver were functioning normally before treatment was started.

The trial with adults followed similar lines. Results from both studies showed that over 50 percent of the patients achieved more than 60 percent improvement in their skin. There was reduced itching but the treatment had no effect on asthma, hayfever or rhinitis. No serious side effects were found.

Patients who took part in the original study were followed up for more than a year. It appears that as long as the treatment continues, the eczema remains inactive with most of the patients for whom it originally worked. After several months some people were able to come off the treatment without the eczema getting any worse and others could have the dose reduced.

What needs to be borne in mind is that the patients who took part in the trials were carefully selected and experienced a particular type of atopic eczema. The formulation used in the trial has not been tested on other types of eczema. Not everyone found that the treatment worked, but everyone hated the taste of the brew.

The standardised herbal brew formulated by Dr Luo still exists in its tea bag form and is marketed under the name of *Zemaphyte* by a pharmaceutical company called Phytopharm Ltd. Although theoretically it can be obtained on prescription this is not easy to come by. It is now only available on prescription by a dermatologist, and this has to be one who believes that Chinese herbal medicine works and will work for you. G.P.s are not permitted to prescribe it for the present. You can obtain it on a private prescription which could be very expensive. This is because *Zemaphyte* does not have a full product licence.

In addition to all this it is unlikely that an NHS prescription would be forthcoming unless routine tests were undertaken. The recommendations for these tests is that a full blood count and routine clinical chemistry tests, including liver function tests, should be taken before starting treatment. These should be repeated regularly throughout the duration of the treatment – after one month, three months and six months and thereafter six-monthly intervals.

This treatment should not be taken by anyone with a known liver or kidney disease, pregnant women or nursing mothers.

There are many clinics in the U.K. offering traditional Chinese herbal medicine. These do not use *Zemaphyte*. Practitioners mix their own brew for patients on an individual basis. Although it is not known exactly how the treatment works, it is thought that the herbal mixture incudes some powerful drugs many of which may be unknown in the West. Just because a treatment is 'natural' does not mean that it is not harmful. There are a small number of Chinese doctors in this country who have been trained in Chinese herbal medicine, but anyone can set up in a practice and it can be difficult to find out whether or not they have the relevant qualifications. So embarking on the treatment in this way can be risky. Death from liver failure of a patient taking Chinese herbal treatment for eczema has been reported, and minor abnormalities of liver function have been detected. You should certainly make sure that you do not undergo this treatment without the regular tests already described. Addresses appear in Chapter 17.

· *Evening primrose oil* ·

This is a naturally occurring oil which appears in the seeds of the evening primrose plant. It is a useful treatment for atopic eczema because it can lessen the itch and improve the health of the skin.

To maintain a healthy body we need to have a balanced diet which has to include a group of nutrients known as essential fatty acids. One particular fatty acid, linoleic acid, is converted by the body into Gamma-linoleic Acid. GLA is needed by the body to maintain a healthy skin and a lack of it can make the skin dry, itchy and scaly.

Normally, obtaining sufficient amounts of essential fatty acids in the diet is not a problem. However, it has been found that some people with atopic eczema are less able to convert the linoleic acid into GLA and this could be a reason for the problem with the skin. Introducing GLA itself into the body seems to be a good option and as evening primrose oil is rich in GLA, taking sufficient quantities of it by mouth is likely to increase its presence in the body.

Trials have found that evening primrose oil can improve the skin of some adults and children with atopic eczema by reducing the itch and the inflammation, but it doesn't work for everybody.

There are many different makes of evening primrose oil available through health shops and pharmacists. However, the brand *Epogam* has been given a product licence. The manufacturers of this brand have carried out tests to check the product's safety. In addition, the particular variety of the evening primrose plant used for this product is grown in controlled conditions to ensure that the oil is pure and that the amount of GLA present remains constant.

Evening primrose oil can be taken safely by most people. However anyone who has epilepsy or is taking medication to prevent fits should not take this treatment. If you are very keen to try it, you must check with your doctor first. He or she will need to keep an eye on you when you start the treatment. Anyone with a history of mental illness or anyone taking any medicine that belongs to the *phenothiazine* group will need to check with their G.P.s before taking evening primrose oil. If you are pregnant or planning on becoming pregnant, speak to your doctor first.

Recommended dosage is 480mg GLA a day for adults and 320mg GLA a day for children. It is *not* suitable for children under a year old.

· *Homoeopathy* ·

The word 'homeo' is Greek and it means 'like'. Homoeopathy is the practice of treating like with like. Not such an extraordinary view when you consider the theory of the 'hair of the dog' or vaccinations and inoculations where you are given a little bit of the very thing you do not want to get!

Homoeopathy was invented in the 18th century by a doctor called Samuel Hahnemann. He felt that traditional medicine had serious shortcomings and he believed that human beings had a capacity for healing themselves. The symptoms of a disease, he thought, were a reflection of a person's struggle to overcome harmful forces; the doctor's work should be to discover, and if possible, remove the cause of the problem and to stimulate the vital healing force of nature.

Dr Hahnemann and his followers carried out experiments on themselves. Over long periods they took small doses of known poisonous or medicinal substances, carefully noting the symptoms they produced (these experiments were called Provings). Patients suffering from similar symptoms were then treated with these substances with good results.

The next step was to establish the smallest effective dose in order to avoid side effects. To his amazement Hahnemann found that, using a special method of dilution, the more the similar remedy was diluted, the more active it became. He called this method *potentisation*. However, this paradox, that less of a substance could be more effective, was not at all acceptable to scientific thought at the time. Hahnemann and his followers were ridiculed.

Today, homoeopathy is a very much respected and a widely used form of medical treatment. The principles are still those established by Hahnemann. The patient is treated – not the disease, so the doctor aims to get a multidimensional picture of the patient.

Remedies are prepared from animal, vegetable and mineral sources. They are diluted, using the process of potentisation that Hahnemann discovered, so that the patient receives an infinitesimal dose of the remedy which, paradoxically, achieves the maximum effect.

The British Homoeopathic Association can give you more information on this treatment and holds a register of homoeopathic doctors. Some G.P.s practise it in their surgeries and there are hospitals in various parts of the country that offer homoeopathy on the NHS.

· *Reflexology* ·

This is a process based on applying pressure to minute areas on the feet. Each zone of the foot correlates to a different part of the body – limbs as well as internal organs. By applying pressure on the soles of the feet it is thought that stress-related illnesses can be helped. This may come about, it is thought, by releasing *endorphins*, morphine-like chemicals in the brain. Also, if the patient feels pain when the therapist is massaging a certain zone in the foot, it may reveal problems in the correlating part of the body. It is a very relaxing and soothing treatment and its contribution in reducing stress in the body can be of benefit to people with eczema.

· *Shiatsu* ·

Again with Shiatsu one of the main benefits is to promote deep relaxation and relief from stress. Shiatsu is a Japanese word which means 'finger pressure'. The theory behind Shiatsu is very similar to that of acupuncture in that the person stays healthy when the flow of energy circulates unimpeded around the body. Pressure is applied to various parts of the body which correspond with the meridians used in acupuncture. The Shiatsu practitioner can apply pressure on the meridian by using his or her thumbs and fingers or elbows and sometimes even knees and feet. This apparently stimulates circulation and the flow of lymphatic fluid. It works on the autonomic nervous system, helps release toxins and tensions from the muscles and can also stimulate the hormonal system. The treatment also enables the patient to relax completely and get in touch with the body's own healing abilities.

Treatment usually starts with a diagnostic session when the practitioner will examine the person's face which, they say, gives a great deal of information about the state of health. Blemishes, lines and colour changes all tell tales to the Shiatsu practitioner. Touch is extensively used as a diagnostic tool and the timbre of the voice is also thought to be an indication of a person's health. 'Hara' diagnosis is sometimes used in which the abdomen is gently palpitated to find out the energetic quality and balance of the various internal organs. Shiatsu practitioners can also diagnose from the pulse.

Shiatsu is complementary to orthodox medicine and practitioners will often give advice on diet and exercise. The length, frequency and total number of sessions varies from person to person.

Since Shiatsu is considered to be so good at relieving stress, if you feel that your eczema is stress-related, it may be worth a try.

· *Transcendental meditation* ·

Many people, including several hundred doctors in the U.K., practise meditation to control stress and promote energy and good health. There are many different techniques you can learn, of which one of the easiest and most readily available is Transcendental Meditation. A great deal of research has gone into TM and it seems that many of the claims made by TM's inventor, Maharishi Mahesh Yogi, and his followers, are not unfounded.

The technique is not at all difficult to master. In a one-to-one session you are given a special sound or phrase called a *mantra*. You shut your eyes, quieten your mind and focus on the mantra. This helps get rid of all the little thoughts that race across the mind. Eventually you let go of the mantra and achieve a deep sense of stillness and inner quiet. The meditating sessions last between fifteen and twenty minutes, but the feeling of peace stays with you, to some extent, throughout the day. As you become a regular meditator – and you are supposed to do it twice a day – this inner peaceful feeling is constantly replenished and emphasised.

For a stress-related condition like eczema, meditation has a very special place. Research has discovered that while sleep triggers the body's restorative powers, the deeper state of the mental relaxation achieved during meditation allows this repair work and recuperation to be carried out more efficiently.

Learning the technique is expensive but it is a one-off payment that lasts for life. Subsequent check-ups, if you need them, are free. It is a seven-stage course which you can learn in about a week.

16

NATIONAL ECZEMA SOCIETY

At Christmas 1975 Christine Orton wrote an article in the *Guardian* newspaper about her son's eczema. "Think of dozens of gnat bites all over your body, in your hair, on your legs, around your eyes, between your fingers – burning, irritating, scratched raw," she wrote. "Then you get somewhere near what the eczema sufferer often puts up with night and day, year in and year out." She ended her article asking: "Perhaps we should form a society for eczema sufferers and their families?"

Within days of the article being published Christine was deluged with letters from people who shared the experiences that she had written about. Two months later Christine and her husband, Peter, organised a meeting at the Bloomsbury offices of the National Council for Voluntary Organisations. Some 80 people attended and a steering committee was formed. Nine months later the National Eczema Society was launched with the broad aim: 'To improve the quality of life for people with eczema and their carers.' Within a year there were local groups all over the country and the Society's magazine *Exchange* was born.

Today the Society is still run by someone who knows about eczema at the sharp end. Tina Funnell first joined the National Eczema Society 15 years ago because her son, Tom, then aged two, had severe eczema. Tina, who started by helping out on an ad hoc basis, became more and more involved.

Her first key job was in organising the National Eczema Society holidays. In 1982, BBC Children in Need Appeal gave the Society funding for a holiday project. There was no one around to run it except for Tina, who had graduated in Social Administration and was currently a full-time youth worker, so she started the holidays and ran the project until 1991. The holidays, which are described in Chapter 10, have since become one of the key on-going projects of the Society and a turning point in the lives of many members – children and adult. Many long-term friendships have developed as a result of the holidays and, not only do some holiday makers from the early holidays still keep in touch with the staff at the national office, but they have so far clocked up two marriages, two partnerships and many long-term friendships.

Tina became General Secretary in 1985 and was appointed Director in 1990.

One of the best ways to improve the quality of life of people with illness is to provide a constant flow of accurate information to patients, carers and the population in general. The National Eczema Society publishes a wide variety of leaflets which effectively do just that. The concept of the core pack of leaflets was devised by a group of mothers attending a public meeting on eczema. The women discussed all the things they felt they needed to know to manage their children's conditions. They also looked at the members' letters and compiled a list of all the points that they felt needed to be mentioned or clarified.

They then set about finding doctors to write some guidelines. At first this was difficult. Medical reticence was such that they were given all sorts of reasons why this couldn't be written and that couldn't be said. But the women stuck to their guns and insisted that what patients needed was clear, practical advice tailored as much as possible to individual needs. And eventually some very informative leaflets were written by leading dermatologists. Today there is a wide variety of leaflets available which target not only the different age groups and environmental situations but also address all the various aspects of living with eczema.

Although the Society has grown from a small handful of caring amateurs to a highly professional and caring team covering education, information, fundraising and management, the core value of putting the patient's view first is still paramount. The problems remain the same too, however, and one of these is getting people to take skin disease seriously. Despite the huge number of patients, dermatology gets few NHS resources. The National Eczema Society relies totally on members' subscriptions, donations and fundraising.

A problem may be that skin diseases are not perceived to claim lives, yet people with eczema herpeticum can die and skin cancer is increasing more rapidly than any other cancer.

Another problem is that the quality of life of some people with eczema can be so bad that they cannot help out on fundraising functions which charities like the National Eczema Society are so reliant upon. Tina Funnell explains:

> If you're living with a chronic condition, especially one that is as painful and as invasive as severe eczema, it affects the whole family. If you've got eczema you feel uncomfortable. You may have social problems if you've got eczema on your face. You may not be able to work if you've got it on your hands. It tends to be much more invasive for a much milder version of the illness than in other chronic conditions. So members may not be able to work for you. They can just about cope with leading their lives without doing the fundraising and awareness of the disease which benefit many other medical charities.

Over the years money has been constantly donated for research into the disease and currently there are six different research projects being funded. The head office in London has a general information service as well as two information lines, one specifically covering Chinese medicinal treatments and the other the use of topical steroids.

The society has also, of course, been extremely active in keeping the needs of eczema patients constantly in the minds of the government, the medical profession and the world at large. They have recently invited other patient groups to work with them to set up a Skin Care Campaign and they now work close with MPs and Peers.

They have also launched a new and very innovative education scheme for the primary health care team. It is novel in that the patient is very much involved. The Society feels that this is necessary with a chronic condition which has no known cure but a variety of different kinds of management.

So along with the modules for doctors and nurses covering the management, care and practical aspects of the illness, comes the patient, in person, giving his side of the story. The patient may explain that what is needed from the medical team is not just a prescription but long-term support and an understanding that it is an illness that affects the whole family. As Tina says:

A doctor may think that a mum is neurotic and not realise that she is exhausted because she is not able to have a full night's sleep. Patients and their carers assume doctors know all about these problems. In fact, if they are not told there is no reason why they should know and understand every aspect of all chronic long-term conditions. So our approach is about explaining to the health care professionals that people with chronic disorders need a different approach to someone whose problem will be solved by an operation.

This scheme, which has been in operation for about a year, is proving very successful.

However, at the end of the day, Tina Funnell reckons that the Society's highest achievement has been to stay in touch with people with eczema and represent their views. "We always put them first," she says. "We know that that's what we're here to do."

The Address of the National Eczema Society is:

4 Tavistock Place
London WC1H 9RA

The NES information line on Chinese medicinal plants and the use of steroids operates from 2pm to 5pm Monday to Friday on 071-388 4800.

17

USEFUL ADDRESSES

Chapter 4

The British Goat Society
34–36 Fore Street
Bovey Tracey
Newton Abbot
Devon TQ13 9AD
Tel: 0626 833168

The Sheep Dairying Association
Wield Wood
Nr Alresford
Hants SO24 9RV
Tel: Alton (0420) 63151

Chapter 5

Pilgrims School
Firle Road
Seaford
East Sussex BN25 2HX
0323 892697

Chapter 9

The National Eczema Society has
several addresses for suppliers of
cotton goods and house dust
mites covers.

Chapter 10

National Eczema Society
4 Tavistock Place
London WC1H 9RA
071-713 0377

National Asthma Campaign
Providence House
Providence Place
London N1 0NT
071-226 2260
Helpline 0345 010203
Mon–Fri 2pm–5pm

Chapter 11

POLY DOTS
Poly (UK) Ltd
10 Allenby Road
Maidenhead
Berks SL6 5BB
0628 33201

SATRA
SATRA House
Rockingham Road
Kettering
Northants NN16 9JH
0536 410000

Chapter 12

NES Information Line
071-388 4800
Mon–Fri 2pm–5pm
Deals specifically with enquiries
on use of topical steroids and
Chinese herbal treatments.

Chelsea and Westminster
Hospitals
369 Fulham Road
London SW10 9NH
081-846 6053

Chapter 14

British Association of
Psychotherapists
37 Mapesbury Road
London NW2 4HJ
081-452 9823

British Association for
Counselling
1 Regent Place
Rugby CV21 2PJ
0788 578328

Relate
Herbert Gray College
Little Church Street
Rugby CV21 3AP
0788 573241

Institute for Transactional
Analysis
BM Box 4104
London WC1N 3XX
071 404 5011

Association of Clinical
Hypnotherapists
229A Sussex Gardens
Lancaster Gate
London W2 2RL
071-402 9037

British Hypnosis Research
Burleigh Business Centre
52 Burleigh Street
Cambridge CB1 1DJ
0223 350012

Elaine Sheehan
1 Well House Court
Well House Road
Oakwood
Leeds LS8 4BS
0532 491073

Chapter 15

British Acupuncture Association
34 Alderney Street
London SW1
071-834 1012/6229

Register of Chinese Herbal
Medicine
21 Warbeck Road
London W12 8NS

Institute of Complementary
Medicine
PO Box 194
London SE16 1QZ
071-237 5165

British Homoeopathic
Association
27A Devonshire Street
London W1N 1RJ
071-935 2163

British School of Reflexology
92 Sheering Road
Old Harlow
Essex CM17 0JW
0279 429060

Shiatsu Society
5 Foxcote
Wokingham
Berks RG11 3PG
0734 730836

Transcendental Meditation
Freepost
London SW1P 4YY
0800 269 303 (Freephone)

INDEX